Baillière's
CLINICAL
PAEDIATRICS
INTERNATIONAL PRACTICE AND RESEARCH

Baillière's
CLINICAL
PAEDIATRICS
INTERNATIONAL PRACTICE AND RESEARCH

Volume 3/Number 2
May 1995

Asthma

P. D. PHELAN BSc, MD, BS, FRACP
Guest Editor

Baillière Tindall
London Philadelphia Sydney Tokyo Toronto

This book is printed on acid-free paper.

Baillière Tindall
W. B. Saunders
Company Ltd

24–28 Oval Road,
London NW1 7DX

The Curtis Center, Independence Square West,
Philadelphia, PA 19106–3399, USA

55 Horner Avenue
Toronto, Ontario M8Z 4X6, Canada

Harcourt Brace & Company
Australia
30–52 Smidmore Street, Marrickville, NSW 2204, Australia

Harcourt Brace & Company
Japan Inc,
Ichibancho Central Building, 22–1
Ichibancho, Chiyoda-ku, Tokyo 102, Japan

ISSN 0963–6714

ISBN 0–7020–1986–0 (single copy)

Baillière's Clinical Paediatrics is published four times each year by Baillière Tindall.
Prices for Volume 3 (1995) are:

TERRITORY	ANNUAL SUBSCRIPTION	SINGLE ISSUE
Europe including UK	£86.00 (Institutional) post free £74.00 (Individual) post free	£30.00 post free
All other countries	Consult your local Harcourt Brace & Company office for dollar price	

The editor of this publication is Gail Greensmith, Baillière Tindall,
24–28 Oval Road, London NW1 7DX.

Typeset by Phoenix Photosetting, Chatham.
Printed and bound in Great Britain by the University Printing House, Cambridge.

Contributors to this issue

GLENN BOWES MBBS, PhD, FRACP, Director, Centre for Adolescent Health, The Royal Children's Hospital and Professor of Adolescent Health, The University of Melbourne, 2 Gatehouse Street, Parkville, Victoria 3052, Australia.

JOHAN C. DE JONGSTE MD, PhD, Associate Professor of Paediatric Respiratory Medicine; Head, Division of Pediatric Respiratory Medicine, Erasmus University and University Hospital, Sophia Children's Hospital, Dr. Molewaterplein 60, 3015 GD Rotterdam, The Netherlands.

DANIEL M. HUGHES BSc, MD, FRCPC, Assistant Professor, Department of Pediatrics, Dalhousie University; Head, Division of Respirology, Izaak Walton Kilam Hospital for Children, 5850 University Avenue, Halifax, Nova Scotia, B3J 3G9 Canada.

ALAN F. ISLES MBBS (Hons), MSc, FRACP, FRCP(C), Associate Professor (Clinical), Paediatric Respiratory Physician, Royal Children's Hospital, Herston, Brisbane, Australia.

JAVIER MALLOL MD, Professor of Pediatrics, Head of Respiratory Medicine, Faculty of Medical Sciences, University of Santiago de Chile, Hospital el Pino, Casilla 40, San Bernardo, Santiago, Chile.

FERNANDO D. MARTINEZ MD, Associate Professor of Pediatrics, University of Arizona College of Medicine, Tucson, AZ 85724, USA.

CHRISTOPHER J. L. NEWTH MB, FRCP(C), FRACP, Director, Division of Pediatric Critical Care, Los Angeles Children's Hospital, 4650 Sunset Boulevard, Los Angeles, CA 90027; Professor of Pediatrics, University of Southern California School of Medicine, Los Angeles, CA, USA.

ANTHONY OLINSKY MBBCH, Dip. Paed., FCPSA, FRACP, Director, Department of Thoracic Medicine, Royal Children's Hospital, Parkville, Victoria 3052, Australia.

HELMUT OSWALD MD, Fellow, Department of Paediatrics, Royal Children's Hospital, Parkville, Victoria 3052, Australia.

SHEILA J. PARK MBChB, MRCPsych, Consultant Psychiatrist and Team Leader; Specialist Medicine Liaison, Mental Health Service, Royal Children's Hospital, Parkville, Victoria 3052, Australia.

PETER D. PHELAN BSc MD, BS, FRACP, Stevenson Professor and Head, Department of Paediatrics, University of Melbourne; Chief Thoracic Physician, Royal Children's Hospital, Parkville, Victoria 3052, Australia.

JOHN F. PRICE MBBCh, MA, MD, FRCP, DCH, Professor of Paediatric Respirology and Consultant Paediatrician, King's College Medical School, Denmark Hill, London SE5 9RS, UK.

K. RAJESHWAR RAO MRCP(Paediatrics), Senior Registrar in Child Health, Southampton General Hospital, Tremona Road, Southampton SO16 6YD, UK.

CHRISTIAN H. L. RIEGER MD, Professor of Pediatrics, Chairman and Director, Klinik für Kinder-und Jugendmedizin der Ruhr-Universität, St. Josef-Hospital, Alexadrinenstrasse 5, 44712 Bochum, Germany.

COLIN F. ROBERTSON MBBS, MSc(Epi), FRACP, Deputy Director, Department of Thoracic Medicine, Royal Children's Hospital, Parkville, Victoria 3054, Australia.

R. G. GARY RUIZ BSc, MBBS, MRCP, Consultant Paediatrician, Department of Child Health, King's College, Denmark Hill, London SE5 9RS, UK.

FELIX H. SENNHAUSER MD, Professor Dr, Head, Pediatric Pulmonology, Ostschweizerisches Kinderspital, Claudiusstrasse 6, CH-9006 St. Gallen; Consultant Respiratory Physician, University Children's Hospital, Zürich, Switzerland.

JOHN O. WARNER MD, FRCP, DCH, Professor of Child Health and Honorary Consultant Paediatrician, University of Southampton, Southampton General Hospital, Tremona Road, Southampton SO16 6YD, UK.

Table of contents

Preface

Asthma is one of the most common conditions leading to a child presenting to either a family doctor or a paediatrician or being admitted to hospital.
Considerable advances in the understanding of asthma have occurred over
recent years. For complex reasons, these have not been matched by
improvements in management. There is substantial evidence that in many
western countries there is overtreatment of children with relatively trivial
asthma, yet those with more troublesome disease often are undertreated.

Therefore it is very appropriate that this issue of *Baillière's Clinical
Paediatrics* be devoted to childhood asthma. It has been possible to bring
together a group of authors who are acknowledged authorities in their
particular field. They have written clearly on important aspects of childhood asthma. Hopefully, this book will be of value to paediatricians, junior
hospital staff and family medical practitioners. It should assist them in their
day to day management of children with asthma.

P. D. PHELAN

1

Asthma in children and adolescents. An overview

PETER D. PHELAN

Asthma is a major health problem for children and adolescents. In many developed countries it is the most frequent cause of long-term health impairment and there is substantial evidence that its prevalence is increasing in many developing countries. While there are health problems of much greater importance in the developing countries, such as malnutrition, low immunization rates, acute gastrointestinal infection and acute respiratory infection, asthma is recognized as requiring particular management strategies appropriate to their social, cultural and economic resources.

THE PREVALENCE OF ASTHMA

There is considerable variation in the prevalence of asthma which is not simply due to the different methodologies used to measure it as discussed by Robertson, et al in Chapter 2. A major concern is the now overwhelming evidence that the prevalence of asthma has increased substantially in many developed countries over the last 10–20 years and it is increasing in developing countries. The reasons for this increase are quite obscure and most explanations offered cannot be supported by available data. The hypothesis that it may be due to some change in allergen exposure is in many ways an attractive one, but at this time unproven. Some enthusiasts are recommending widespread intervention programs to reduce allergen exposure without these being tested on a scientifically rigorous basis. As management of so much human disease is based on impression and anecdote, it would be a tragedy if we could not design double-blind controlled clinical trials to demonstrate that these proposed interventions are efficacious and have a very positive cost benefit. Christian Rieger in Chapter 9 provides a comprehensive overview of the current state of knowledge of the relationship of allergy to asthma and indicates where many of the challenges lie.

Baillière's Clinical Paediatrics—
Vol. 3, No. 2, May 1995
ISBN 0–7020–1986–0

UNDERTREATMENT OR OVERTREATMENT

Despite the publication of a number of international consensus statements on the management of asthma in children, there continues to be substantial evidence for overtreatment of those whose asthma is a relatively trivial health problem and undertreatment of those whose lifestyles is substantially interfered by it (Rosier et al, 1994). There are probably many complex reasons for why this parodoxical situation has arisen.

Over the last 10–15 years there has been increasing recognition that the basic pathology of asthma is airways inflammation and that airways obstruction as a result of smooth muscle spasm is a secondary phenomenon. Most of the evidence for this has come from bronchial biopsies undertaken in adults and the application of this data to children is discussed by Rao and Warner in Chapter 3.

The emphasis on inflammation as the pathology of asthma has led to suggestions that it is imperative to treat this inflammation to alter the natural history of asthma and to prevent the development of irreversible airways disease (Agertoft and Pedersen, 1994). While again this is an attractive suggestion, epidemiological studies of the natural history of asthma and the few long-term studies of effective treatment, do not give much support to it. Over half the children with relatively infrequent episodes of asthma will become wheeze-free in early adult life irrespective of any treatment (Martin et al, 1981). While the asthma resolves, allergic features may become more marked, again questioning the interrelationship between asthma and other manifestations of allergy. Irreversible airways disease is a very rare phenomenon in mid adult life, even in those who have had airways obstruction for nearly 30 years as discussed in Chapter 3. Whether it will develop in later adult life is not known and must await further long-term studies. The contribution of tobacco smoking to the irreversible airways disease seen in some adults with asthma (Brown et al, 1984) may be of critical importance. Regrettably too many children and adolescents with asthma are regular smokers. The one moderately long-term study of the use of corticosteroids failed to show any long-term benefit in those in whom the drug was ceased after 2–3 years (van Essen-Zandvliet et al, 1992).

Probably the most single important reason for the undertreatment of those with persistent asthma and the overtreatment of those with trivial asthma has been the failure to define precisely the severity of the disorder. The way terms are used can create confusion in the minds of primary health care providers and of parents. In Chapter 5 Phelan et al suggest a precise definition of the severity of acute episodes and of the degree of lifestyle impairment in the long-term, based on the frequency of acute episodes and the presence of interval symptoms. These guidelines may provide a useful basis for decisions about therapy.

Parental anxiety often compounded by physician anxiety may lead to the overtreatment of relatively trivial asthma when severity is not appropriately defined. A family's reaction to illness is a major influence on the treatment given. In Chapter 11 Sheila Park discusses many aspects of the family psychodynamics in asthma. While she is referring particularly to a group with obvious emotional problems, if adequate explanations are not given to parents and adolescents about asthma, its nature, its natural history and likely impact on lifestyle, then undoubtedly anxiety will continue and excess treatment will probably be used. Conversely there are some families who seem to deny the presence of illness and they and their child with troublesome persistent asthma accept the child's persistent symptoms and impaired lifestyle as normal. Unless their physician asks the appropriate questions such as the frequency of wheeze, whether nights are disturbed by asthma, the number of times a β_2 agent needs to be used during the day, then the presence of persistent troublesome asthma will be missed. The failure to measure lung function or reliance simply on the measurement of peak flow which may miss troublesome airways obstruction completely exacerbates the problem. Ruiz and Price in Chapter 6 give clear guidelines as to the role of lung function measurements in the management of asthma.

The use of peak flow meters in childhood asthma in particular needs re-evaluation as discussed in Chapter 6. They are very effort-dependent and substantial numbers of children are being seen who are receiving excessive doses of inhaled corticosteroids on the basis of falsely low measurements of peak flow. It may be that more children with asthma are genuinely harmed because their treatment is based on peak flow measurements, than are helped by such measurements over and above what can be adduced from history and physical examination. Because there is a figure, it does not mean that this reflects reality.

Many of the treatment plans for asthma have been developed by adult chest physicians and then extrapolated to children. It seems probable that the majority of adults with asthma seen by chest physicians fall into the group of persistent asthma as defined by Phelan et al in Chapter 5 and the treatment plans have been directed to this group. For a period it was thought that this was the predominant pattern of asthma in adults but recent epidemiological studies (Abramson et al, 1992) have indicated that the patterns of frequent episodic asthma and infrequent episodic asthma do occur in adults. However, patients with these may not seek medical advice or if they do they rarely progress beyond primary care. Many adults are excellent at denying the significance of minor respiratory symptoms and fail to seek medical attention. If a child wheezes then his mother is likely to become anxious and will seek medical advice whereas if she or her husband has similar symptoms they may well do nothing about them. This is frequently seen in paediatric practice when a history is taken of illnesses from parents. All too often one is told that 'my husband gets wheezy when he has a cold or when he plays sport but he doesn't need to do anything about it' by an anxious mother who presents with a child who has two or three episodes of wheeze a year associated with intercurrent viral infections. The classification of asthma into infrequent episodic, frequent episodic, and persistent is being used increasingly by adult chest physicians as a useful one. This will probably lead to different treatment plans to those now promoted for adults.

A group with wheeze in the paediatric age group who seem to be frequently overtreated are those in the first 1–2 years of life. The work by

Martinez et al in Tucson, Arizona, as reviewed in Chapter 4, has demonstrated that only about one in three infants with minor episodes of wheeze really have asthma. Regrettably there are no predictive features that would allow one to say with absolute confidence which wheezy episode in an infant or young child is asthma and which is viral infection-induced wheeze because of narrowing of already small airways. Certainly this work has reinforced the importance of not overtreating such infants either with bronchodilators or, more importantly, with prophylactic drugs which may have quite significant side effects. The whole question of the management of the wheezy infant needs careful re-evaluation in terms of this new information.

MANAGEMENT STRATEGIES

The goals of the management of asthma are:

(i) to achieve rapid resolution of acute episodes, to relieve respiratory distress and to prevent the episodes being a threat to wellbeing or life; and

(ii) to allow the child or adolescent and his/her family to enjoy a normal lifestyle by the use, where appropriate, of prophylactic drugs ensuring their benefit is not outweighed by side effects, which include simply the need to take medication two to three times a day.

Isles and Newth comprehensively review in Chapter 7 the treatment of acute episodes of asthma and they provide a most valuable flow chart for the treatment of acute episodes. Response to treatment following their guidelines complements the definition of acute episodes given by Phelan et al in Chapter 3. De Jongste in Chapter 8 comprehensively reviews prophylactic drugs and suggests very sensible guidelines for their use. These are very consistent with the classification suggested by Phelan et al so that those children with infrequent episodic asthma do not require prophylactic therapy. In those with frequent episodic asthma, sodium cromoglycate would generally be the choice for initial therapy while inhaled corticosteroids would be required by the majority of patients with persistent asthma, although in those at the less troubled end of this group, sodium cromoglycate may be effective. De Jongste makes the interesting suggestion, which should be carefully evaluated, that perhaps rapid control of frequent episodic asthma by the use of inhaled corticosteroids and then substituting sodium cromoglycate would be a better approach than the more widely used current one of gradually increased therapy if symptoms are not controlled. The rapid gain of confidence of parents in seeing their child's symptoms controlled with a short period of inhaled corticosteroids would be extremely beneficial provided inertia did not lead to the continuation of inhaled corticosteroids when the child would be equally well controlled on sodium cromoglycate. The total absence of side effects in the latter in contrast to the albeit quite occasional side effects from the former should encourage its use when it controls symptoms.

Many parents look to non-pharmacological approaches for the control of their child's asthma. Regrettably there is virtually no evidence that any of these have any benefit. Breathing exercises and physiotherapy have been tried for many years and despite claims of benefit, these are not supported by adequate clinical trials. Allergen avoidance is an attractive approach, but is not easy as discussed by Rieger in Chapter 9. While simple measures to avoid housedust mite may be of some help, they are rarely dramatic. Whether or not intensive allergen avoidance in the early months of life, in those with risk factors for the development of asthma, will prove to be effective can only be determined on the basis of proper clinical trials.

Parents often turn to alternative health care providers when traditional medicine appears to fail to control their child's symptoms or because of their anxiety, usually unwarranted, about side effects of pharmacological agents. The fact that they seek this advice is usually a reflection of the failure of their physicians to communicate accurately to parents and families the nature of asthma, the goals of therapy and the great safety of most of the medications used for asthma.

The importance of managing asthma in adolescents in terms of the developmental stage is stressed by Glenn Bowes in Chapter 10. For treatment to be successful, the appropriate regime must be negotiated with the teenager and what is considered ideal therapy should be adjusted to be in keeping with the young person's lifestyle, educational and career goals.

EDUCATION

A whole industry is developing around asthma education programmes and these are comprehensively reviewed in Chapter 12 by Dan Hughes. While many of these programmes increase the knowledge of asthma, there is scanty evidence that they improve overall management. Certainly very few of them have been subject to a proper cost benefit analysis.

Hughes rightly emphasizes the primacy of education about asthma given by the treating physician to the parents, child and adolescent. Precise information about what drugs are to be used, when they are to be used and their possible side effects is essential if management is to be appropriate. Wherever possible these guidelines should be given in written form and in very simple terms. For the vast majority of children, management plans based on symptoms are more likely to be helpful than those based on measurement of peak flow. Particularly during acute episodes of asthma, peak flow measurements in children may be quite unreliable.

It is a tragedy to see the continuing morbidity in children and adolescents because of inappropriate treatment of asthma and the failure to deal with many of the anxieties associated with the disease which in themselves can result in morbidity—so-called prescribed morbidity. The unnecessary use of prophylactic medication two or three times a day in children with infrequent episodic asthma simply reinforces to the child and family that he has a significant health problem which is not so. With proper explanation and education of patient and family and the use in the vast majority of children and adolescents with asthma of no more than two pharmacological agents, the morbidity from the disease should be readily controlled.

SUMMARY

Many of the important topics in childhood and adolescent asthma are discussed in the following chapters which hopefully will be of assistance to family practitioners, paediatricians and hospital staff involved in the care of children and adolescents. Scientific information is provided that is the essential basis of a logical management plan.

REFERENCES

Abramson M, Kutin J & Bowes G (1992) The prevalence of asthma in Victorian adults. *Australian and New Zealand Journal of Medicine* **22:** 358–363.

Agertoft L & Pedersen S (1994) Effects of long term treatment with an inhaled corticosteroid on growth and pulmonary function in asthmatic children. *Respiratory Medicine* **88:** 373–381.

Brown PJ, Greville HW & Finucane Ke (1984) Asthma and irreversible airways obstruction. *Thorax* **39:** 130–136.

Martin AJ, Landau LI & Phelan PD (1981) The natural history of allergy in asthmatic children followed to adult life. *Medical Journal of Australia* **2:** 470–474.

Rosier MJ, Bishop J, Nolan T et al (1994) Measurement of functional severity of asthma in children. *American Journal of Respiratory and Critical Care Medicine* **149:** 1434–1441.

Van Essen-Zandvliet EE, Hughes MD, Waalkens HJ et al (1992) Effects of 22 months of treatment with inhaled corticosteroids and/or beta-2 agonists on lung function, airway responsiveness and symptoms in children with asthma. *American Review of Respiratory Disease* **146:** 547–554.

2

The change in prevalence and severity of asthma in developed and developing countries

COLIN F. ROBERTSON
FELIX H. SENNHAUSER
JAVIER MALLOL

The definition of asthma has been widely debated for many years, with most pathophysiological definitions differing little from that of Scadding (1963), which describes the functional consequences: 'asthma is a disease characterised by wide variations over short periods of time in resistance to flow in intra-pulmonary airways'. While clinicians may agree on this or similar definitions, it is then necessary to adapt such a physiological definition to one more suitable for epidemiological purposes. An epidemiological definition must accurately reflect the disease to be studied, yet its criteria must be able to be met by the data available from the survey. To date, there is no 'gold standard' for the epidemiological definition of asthma and as a result, the definition for epidemiological purposes will differ widely between studies. To allow comparison between studies, it is essential to ensure that the definition used for each study is similar.

The most widely used definition of asthma in children, for epidemiological purposes, is a history of wheeze. In developed, English speaking countries, there is a high level of agreement between a history of wheeze and a clinical diagnosis of asthma. However, such a definition is subject to recall, the level of awareness of symptoms and asthma in the community and a variety of cultural and sociological factors and, therefore, may not necessarily be generalizable to other cultures where either the language or spectrum of respiratory illness is different. In some languages, there is no direct translation for 'wheeze'. In some developing countries, lung disease due to infection is very common and a history of wheeze is unable to distinguish between recurrent respiratory infections and asthma (Flynn, 1994). Recall of symptoms either by an individual or parent can be variable, particularly for events that occurred well in the past. To minimize the effect of variable recall, the period for which the symptoms are asked is usually limited to 12 months.

In some studies, a history of a 'doctor diagnosis' of asthma has been used to determine the prevalence of asthma. Such a definition is subject not only to influence by those factors listed above, but will also be influenced by access to health services and the training of the medical practitioner to

253
Copyright © 1995, by Baillière Tindall

recognize asthma and their readiness to label a child as having asthma with all that may be attached to such a label in some communities. In most studies where 'doctor diagnosis of asthma' has been compared with other symptoms or bronchial reactivity, it has under-represented the prevalence of asthma in that population (Anderson et al, 1983; Speight et al, 1983).

Measures of bronchial responsiveness provide an objective measure of airway abnormality which, although quite specific, are not very sensitive as a test for asthma. Tests using both pharmacological agents such as histamine and methacholine, and non-pharmacological agents, such as hypertonic saline, exercise, cold air and distilled water, have been developed for use in the field (Sears et al, 1986a; Peat et al, 1988; Frischer et al, 1992; Nicolai et al, 1993; Haby et al, 1994; Riedler et al, 1995) and show sensitivities between 31 and 53% with specificities ranging from 88 to 92% (Riedler et al, 1995).

The combination of a history of recent wheeze and bronchial hyperresponsiveness has been suggested as a more robust definition of asthma for epidemiological purposes (Toelle, 1992). This definition, which has low sensitivity is highly specific, identifies the group of children with more severe disease and may allow a more consistent comparison between countries and within countries over time. It also appears to distinguish symptoms due to recurrent respiratory tract infections better than from those due to asthma (Flynn, 1994).

In summary, any universal epidemiological definition for asthma needs to be validated within the community for which it is to be used. The difficulty is to identify a 'gold standard' within that community against which to validate the definition. In Australia, we have used a physician diagnosis of asthma established after interview by a paediatric respiratory physician. As asthma remains a clinical diagnosis, similar strategies may need to be developed for each community.

THE PREVALANCE OF ASTHMA AND ITS VARIATION AROUND THE WORLD

The prevalence of asthma varies widely throughout the world, ranging from less than 1% in some developing countries to more than 25% in some developed countries. When reviewing international prevalance studies, it is necessary to consider the definition used, whether it relies on a reported history of wheeze alone, a doctor diagnosis of asthma or a combination of history of symptoms and bronchial hyperresponsiveness. It is also necessary to consider the period over which the symptoms are recorded, as a lifetime prevalence will be higher than a 12 month period prevalence. Recollection of events beyond 12 months is less reliable, therefore, a 12 month period prevalence of reported symptoms is the accepted standard (ISAAC, 1992). The year in which data for the study was collected should also be considered, as in most countries there has been an increase in prevalence of asthma over time. Age influences the prevalence of asthma and is therefore important to consider when making comparisons. The most common age range studied is 7 to 12-year-old children, over which the prevalence changes little. The prevalence of asthma has been most widely studied in Australia, New Zealand and the United Kingdom. The most recent studies show the prevalence of asthma, defined as 'a history of wheeze in the past 12 months', as 25.4% in Australia (Peat et al, 1994) 18.7% in New Zealand (Mitchell and Asher, 1994) and 15.9% in England (Strachan et al, 1994). However, there is considerable international variation even when differences in methodology are allowed for. Similar high prevalence rates to those reported in Australia and New Zealand have been noted when almost identical questionnaires were used in Chile (Robertson et al, 1993) and Fiji (Flynn, 1994). The prevalence was found to be much lower in Switzerland at 7% (Robertson et al, 1993). In recent years, there have been several studies performed internationally and the results are summarized in Table 1.

Gender differences in the prevalence of asthma are consistent throughout the above studies. There is a male predominance of current asthma in children under the age of 10, and this difference is lost by the early teen years. It has been suggested that one contributing factor is a tendency to under-diagnosis and undertreatment in girls with symptoms suggestive of asthma (Kuhni and Sennhauser, 1995).

There are many factors which may explain the regional variation in prevalence of asthma. Genetic factors have been clearly shown to be important in determining the propensity to asthma. This is best demonstrated in studies of twins where concordance for asthma is much higher in monozygotic twins than dizygotic twins (Edfors-Lubs, 1971; Duffy et al, 1990). Children of asthmatic parents have an increased prevalence of bronchial hyperresponsiveness even in the absence of symptoms of asthma (Clifford et al, 1987). However, the mode of inheritance remains in doubt. Current data would suggest that asthma is the result of polygenetic or multifactorial inheritance.

Regional variations in the prevalence of asthma within a population of the same genetic stock suggest that environmental factors are also important. This has been best demonstrated by the change in prevalence of asthma among those who have migrated from areas of low prevalence to areas of high prevalence where they acquire the higher prevalence of their adopted country. Waite et al (1980) found that asthma prevalence increased more than two-fold in Tokelauan children who migrated to New Zealand compared to those who stayed on the island. Interestingly, Leung et al (1994b) have shown substantial differences in the prevalence of asthma and atopy between Asian immigrants to Australia, Australian-born Asians and Australian-born nonAsians. The prevalence of asthma among Asian-born immigrants was lower than the Australian-born Asians and Australian-born nonAsians and increased with their length of stay in Australia.

The components of environment that influence asthma are not well defined. Air pollution has been commonly promoted as a major contributor to asthma prevalence. However, a recent study from Germany has shown the lifetime prevalence of asthma, the current prevalence of wheezing, atopy and bronchial hyperresponsiveness to be higher in children from

Table 1. Prevalence rates for asthma in children for developed countries.

Country	Age (years)	Current wheeze	Current asthma	Lifetime wheeze	Lifetime asthma	Symptoms and BHR	Reference
Australia	8–10	25.4			31.8	10.5	Peat et al (1994)
Australia	7–8	23.1	18.0	41.0	24.1		Robertson et al (1991)
New Zealand	7–10	18.7		30.1	16.3		Mitchell and Asher (1994)
England	8–10	15.9		23.4	12.6		Strachan et al (1994)
W. Germany	9–11		5.9	17.0	9.3		Von Mutius et al (1994a)
Switzerland	7–8	7.4		18.4	4.3		Robertson et al (1991)
Sweden	10–12	10.6	6.9				Braback et al (1994)
Poland	10–12	10.4	2.9				Braback et al (1994)
United States	8–11	5.4			3.9		Schwartz et al (1990)
Chile	7–8	26.2		50.8	9.4		Robertson et al (1991)
Hong Kong	6–8	6.6		15.4	10.0		Leung et al (1994a)
Fiji	8–10	21.0		25.3	8.4	8.0	Flynn (1994)

Current wheeze: history of wheeze within the last 12 months; Lifetime wheeze: history of wheeze at any time in the child's life; Current asthma: symptoms of asthma within the last 12 months plus a diagnosis of asthma; Lifetime asthma: a diagnosis of asthma at any time in the child's life.

Munich than the polluted cities of Liepzig and Halle in the former East Germany (von Mutius et al, 1994a). In this study there was a higher prevalence of allergic disorders in Munich suggesting that there may be aetiological factors associated with Western lifestyles and living conditions. Two studies of Australian children have recorded similar prevalence rates for asthma and atopy between urban and rural regions (Robertson et al, 1992a; Peat et al, 1994). In these regions, genetic stock and lifestyle were similar but the levels of environmental air pollution were vastly different. One difficulty in examining the relationship between air pollution and asthma lies in the definition of pollution. Those substances currently measured may not be relevant to asthma and relevant thresholds are yet to be defined. The relationship between environmental air pollution and asthma seems more apparent for acute asthma, particularly nitrogen dioxide (Neas et al, 1991) and particulate matter (Pope and Dockery, 1992).

There are several other environmental factors which may influence the prevalence of asthma to be addressed elsewhere. These include environmental allergens such as housedust mite and grass and tree pollens (Sporick et al, 1990; Peat et al, 1993), environmental tobacco smoke (Young et al, 1991; US Environmental Protection Agency, 1992) and diet (Peat et al, 1992a). Asthma may be linked to the total level of allergen load rather than specific allergens. In the Australian studies of urban and rural regions the prevalence rate of both asthma and atopy were similar yet the patterns of specific allergen responses were different. The urban population of Belmont were more likely to be sensitized to housedust mite whereas the rural population in Wagga were more likely to be sensitized to rye grass, pollen and *Alternaria tienius*, an opportunistic mould that proliferates in dead plant material in dry regions (Peat et al, 1994). A French study has also reported similar prevalence rates of respiratory symptoms and atopy between a coastal and an alpine region with prevalence of sensitivity to housedust mite four-fold higher in the coastal region and to grass pollen being three times higher in the alpine region (Sharpin et al, 1991).

EVIDENCE FOR CHANGES BOTH IN PREVALENCE AND SEVERITY OF ASTHMA

In each country where serial measurements have been made, there has been a consistent rise in the prevalence of asthma.

In Australia, studies from the 1960s to 1990s show a consistent increase in the prevalence of lifetime history of wheeze from 19% in 1969 to 41% in 1990 (Robertson et al, 1991). Some 18 studies in asthma prevalence in children aged 5–12 years have been reported between 1969 and 1992. When analysed serially, there has been an average increase in the prevalence of asthma at a rate of 0.7% per annum (Bauman, 1993). Although these studies involve different investigators and populations, the trend was similar when the same team of investigators examined the same population. In Australia there have been three recent serial surveys. A study from New

South Wales (NSW) over 10 years showed a 95% increase in the 12 month period prevalence of wheeze from 13.0% in 1982 to 25.4% in 1992 (Peat et al, 1994). Studies from Melbourne 26 years apart, looking at the lifetime prevalence of wheeze showed an increase of 141% from 19.1% in 1964 to 41% in 1990 (Robertson et al, 1991). A similar study in Tasmania over 24 years showed an increase of 112% in the lifetime prevalence of wheeze from 1964 to 1992 (Jenkins et al, 1994).

Similar trends have been demonstrated in the United Kingdom. In Croydon, a repeat study of 7 to 8-year-old children using the same school age groups and similar questionnaires reported an increase in the 12 month period prevalence of wheeze of 27% over 13 years from 9.7% in 1982 to 12.3% in 1991 (Anderson et al, 1994). In Cardiff, the increase over 15 years was 55% (Burr et al, 1989) and in Aberdeen there was an even higher increase but the questions in each survey for this study were not the same (Ninan and Russell, 1992). Two other British studies have shown similar increases (Burney et al, 1990, Whincup et al, 1993). In North America, a recent Canadian study found a substantial increase in the physician-diagnosed asthma between 1980 and 1990 (Manfreda et al, 1993). In this study, which covered all ages, the greatest increase was seen in children. A study from the United States also reported an increase in the lifetime prevalence of asthma from 4.8% in 1974–1976 to 7.6% in 1980–1984 (Gergen et al, 1988).

Although the serial studies referred to above have used similar method-ology there is a potential error from increased awareness of symptoms within the community and diagnostic transfer. There is now excellent objective evidence to support the increase in reported symptoms. The serial studies in children in NSW carried out 10 years apart included objective measures of bronchial responsiveness to histamine (Peat et al, 1994). In 1982, the prevalence of bronchial hyperresponsiveness to histamine in these children was 9.1% and in 1992 it was 19.8% representing an increase of 117%. Interestingly the prevalence of atopy, which was measured by skin prick testing to common allergens, remained unchanged (28% in 1982, 29% in 1992). The increase in rate of bronchial hyperresponsiveness occurred predominantly in the atopic group of children. A similar study of adults in Western Australia showed the prevalence of bronchial hyper-responsiveness to remain at approximately 10% over a 10 year period (Peat et al, 1992b).

The only other repeat study to include a measure of bronchial respon-siveness was in Welsh children using free-running exercise as the provok-ing stimulus (Burr et al, 1989). In this study, the range of bronchial hyperresponsiveness increased from 6.7% in 1974 to 7.7% in 1988. This was only a modest increase during a period where reported doctor-diagnosed asthma rose from 4 to 9% and atopic dermatitis increased from 5 to 16%.

While the prevalence of asthma has been shown to be increasing consis-tently in several countries, there are conflicting reports about changes in severity. In the United Kingdom comparative study, there was an increase in prevalence but, with the exception of sleep disturbance due to asthma, a paradoxical reduction in chronic disability such as school absence (Anderson et al, 1994). There was no change in the number of severe attacks. This paradox was attributed to improvement in recognition and treatment of asthma within the community. In the serial study in NSW, there appeared to be an increase in asthma severity, as measured by frequency of symptoms, proportional to the increase in prevalence (Peat et al, 1994). Other indices of severity such as hospital admission rates and mortality rates will be discussed below.

There is now clear evidence from several countries, both subjective and objective, of a continuing increase in the prevalence of asthma in children. In addition to an increase in asthma, there have been increases of similar magnitude in the prevalence of other atopic conditions such as eczema and hayfever, but no change in the proportion expressing atopy as measured by skin prick testing with common allergens (Anderson et al, 1994; Peat et al, 1994). Unfortunately there is no clear explanation for such an increase. It is unlikely that the genetic factors could be responsible for such an increase over the relatively short time-frame of one decade. This suggests that a change in some component of the environment is likely to be responsible.

Major candidates for such change include air pollution, both indoor and outdoor, total allergen load, diet and maternal cigarette smoking. The evidence available suggests that the impact of environmental air pollution is greater on those with chronic bronchitis than those with asthma (Oshima et al, 1964). There have been several reports of epidemics of acute asthma in association with periods of high air pollution, but on further examination this has been found to be a result of high airborne allergen load. The best described example is that which occurred in Barcelona in the 1980s. Initially, the epidemic was thought to be due to high levels of nitrogen dioxide. However, further analysis identified high levels of soybean allergen in the air as a result of unusual weather conditions and the loading of soybean in the harbour (Anto et al, 1989). The evidence for an effect of air pollution on the prevalence of asthma is less convincing. The recent study comparing prevalence of asthma between the former East and West Germany showed an inverse relationship between prevalence of asthma and air pollution in a population of identical genetic background (von Mutius et al, 1994a) and several studies in Australia have shown a similar prevalence of asthma in rural and urban environments where the level of pollution is vastly different (Robertson et al, 1992a; Peat et al, 1994). In fact, while the prevalence of asthma is increasing in the United States, the concentration of the major air pollutants has declined substantially over the past 25 years (Lang and Polansky, 1994). There has been a similar fall in air pollution in the United Kingdom following reduction in the burning of coal. The evidence for the impact of indoor air pollutants is inconclusive or shows only minimal effect.

Diet is a potential environmental factor which may influence the development of asthma. The changes in prevalence of asthma seen following migration are likely to be associated with a change in diet. The daily intake of dietary sodium is known to increase with economic development

(Gleibermann, 1973). Some years ago, Burney reported a significant association between the rate of asthma mortality and sales of table salt in
regions of England and Wales. This was found particularly in the 5 to 14-
year-old age group (Burney, 1985). In addition, a high salt intake and a
high 24 hour urinary sodium excretion have been associated with increased
bronchial responsiveness (Burney et al, 1986; Javid, 1988). In the NSW
study, there was also a significant protective effect of diet seen. Children
who ate regular fish meals, more than once a week, were only one-third as
likely to have bronchial hyperresponsiveness as nonfish eaters (Peat et al,
1992a). While fish oil has been shown to impair the production of lipid
mediators and blunt the late allergic response in asthmatics, clinical trials
have failed to demonstrate an improvement in clinical asthma (Arm et al,
1989). Seaton has suggested that host resistance to environmental allergens
has declined because of an alteration in diet associated with 'westernization' of societies (Seaton et al, 1994).

Fetal and early infancy may be a critical period for environmental factors
to influence the prevalence of asthma. The increase in prevalence of asthma
has coincided in an increase in smoking rates in young women. Maternal
smoking has been shown to affect lung development in utero (Young et al,
1991; Hanrahan et al, 1992) and children who are exposed to maternal
smoking are more likely to have respiratory tract infections (Wright et al,
1991) and attend emergency rooms for asthma (Evans et al, 1987). Equally
there appears to be a critical period in early infancy when the genetically
susceptible child may become sensitized to environmental allergens (Holt
et al, 1990). The effect of breast-feeding on the development of asthma has
been widely studied. While there may be some benefit for reduction in the
development of eczema, two large British cohort studies failed to demonstrate any protection of breast-feeding against the development of asthma
(Taylor et al, 1983; Anderson et al, 1986).

The explanation behind the rising of prevalence of asthma is complicated
and remains poorly understood. It is vitally important to have a clearer
understanding of the reasons behind the increase before intervention strategies can be developed.

CHANGING HOSPITAL ADMISSION RATES FOR ASTHMA

The prevalence rates, and hospital admission rates for asthma in children
have increased in several countries, although the increases have not been
parallel. In Australia, asthma is the most common cause for admission to a
paediatric hospital bed accounting for approximately 6% of admissions.
The admission rate has doubled over the past two decades (Kun et al,
1993). Similar changes have been reported from the United Kingdom
(Strachan and Anderson, 1992), New Zealand (Mitchell et al, 1990) and the
United States (Weiss and Wagener, 1990). In each of these countries there
was a dramatic increase during the 1970s which stabilized throughout the
1980s resulting in a negligible increase over that period. There are three
principle explanations for an increase in hospital admissions: an increase in

the prevalence or severity of asthma in the paediatric population; diagnostic transfer from other nonasthma respiratory conditions such as bronchitis; and a change in the pattern of management.

The increase in prevalence of asthma is no doubt a contributing factor, but does not fully account for the increase in hospital admissions. In the United Kingdom, increase in hospital admissions was in excess of the increase in prevalence and over the same time period the pattern of severity appeared to be unchanged. While there has been a dramatic increase in the prevalence of asthma in Australia over those two decades, the increase has been at a constant rate of between 0.7 and 1.0% per annum (Bauman, 1993). The major increase in hospital admission rates occurred during the first of these two decades with little change during the second decade when there was both subjective and objective evidence of a continuing increase in the prevalence of asthma (Peat et al, 1994). In New Zealand, the admission rate increased 10-fold in the 15 years from the mid 1960s (Mitchell, 1985) which was also well in excess of the increase in the prevalence of asthma. There was little change in the admission rate for paediatric asthma during the 1980s.

Reports of the contribution of diagnostic transfer to the reported increase in admission rates have been conflicting. Carmen suggested that the increase in admission rates for paediatric asthma in Western Australia could be accounted for by a proportional reduction in nonasthma respiratory conditions (Carmen and Landau, 1990). However, a similar study in NSW reported a 98% increase in the number of hospital admissions due to asthma without an apparent fall in the number of admissions for nonasthma respiratory conditions (Kun et al, 1993). In the United Kingdom study, twice as many wheezy children had been diagnosed as asthmatic in the 1991 survey compared to the 1978 survey, supporting the influence of a change in diagnostic labelling (Strachen and Anderson, 1992). The same study reported a marked change in utilization of health care services. Over the 13 year period there was more than a two-fold increase in the number reporting to a casualty department for treatment of their acute asthma. There was a corresponding 50% reduction of those reporting treatment of acute asthma by a general practitioner at home. Greater use of the diagnosis of asthma and changing attitudes to the management of acute asthma may underlie the observed shift from general practitioner care to casualty department attendance. A child with mild to moderate asthma who is managed in a casualty department is far more likely to be admitted to hospital than the child being managed at home by the general practitioner. The pattern of health care utilization may also have been influenced by a change in the structure of general practice. There has been a shift away from the traditional family general practitioner to the less personal multiple doctor clinics which may result in less continuity of care.

It is likely that the diagnostic transfer has occurred in the community rather than within the hospital which results in more children seeking management of acute attacks in a hospital casualty department rather than by a general practitioner. This change in health care utilization together with an increase in the prevalence of asthma would account for the increase reported in hospital admission rates due to asthma.

MORTALITY DUE TO ASTHMA IN CHILDREN AND
ADOLESCENTS—IS IT CHANGING AND WHO IS AT RISK?

The interpretation of mortality statistics is dependent on their accuracy. Studies from the United Kingdom, New Zealand and Australia, countries of high asthma prevalence, have shown the official mortality statistics to have reasonable accuracy in the 15- to 64-year-old age group. There was a tendency to overestimation by 12.9% in New Zealand (Sears et al, 1986b), 13.5% in the United Kingdom (British Thoracic Society, 1984) and 12.5% in Australia (Jenkins et al, 1992). The overestimate is much higher in those aged 65 years and over. The accuracy is not so well known for other countries that report a low incidence of asthma mortality where there may be a tendency to under-reporting by these countries (Burney, 1989). Accuracy seems to be highest for the 5- to 34-year-old age group and this group is usually used for international comparisons.

There is a wide variation in asthma mortality rates between countries. While those countries with a higher prevalence of asthma tend to have higher mortality rates, the different medical practices and reporting procedures make interpretation difficult. Although there were two- to three-fold differences in asthma mortality between New Zealand, Canada and Australia, cross-sectional studies of asthma prevalence in children, using the same definition of asthma and measures of bronchial responsiveness, have shown no differences between these countries (Asher et al, 1988; Fitzgerald et al, 1988). Mortality rates for 1990 for countries where they are available are listed in Table 2.

In addition to variation between countries, there are within-country variations reported. In New Zealand, the mortality rate is two- to four-fold higher amongst the Maori population (Sears et al, 1985). In the United States generally, the mortality rate for African Americans is twice that of whites and in the innercity areas, the difference increases to five times (Weiss and Wagener, 1990; Carr et al, 1992). In New York, the rates varied by neighbourhood and correlated significantly with race and poverty. These differences are likely to be a reflection of a tendency to use acute health

Table 2. International mortality rates for asthma in 5 to 34-year-olds for 1990.

Country	Mortality Rate (per 100 000 population)
Australia	1.13
Singapore	1.05
New Zealand	0.79
England/Wales	0.74
Japan	0.69
West Germany	0.56
Switzerland	0.50
USA	0.43
Canada	0.37
France	0.37
Austria	0.32

care facilities more commonly and to have limited access to prophylactic management, both of which have been shown to be significant risk factors for asthma mortality (Rea et al, 1986).

Variation over time

Time trends in asthma mortality can also be affected by changes in definition and changes in medical practice which may influence coding practice. Asthma mortality had been relatively stable throughout the first half of this century until the 1960s. During the 1960s there was a sharp two- to three-fold increase in mortality rates reported from the United Kingdom, New Zealand and Australia, with no change reported from other countries (Figure 1). The cause of this epidemic, which had resolved by the end of the decade, has been attributed to the introduction of a high dose preparation of isoprenaline which was five times the strength of the previously available metered dose inhaler (Speizer et al, 1968; Inman and Adelstein, 1969).

Since then, there has been a gradual but consistent increase in mortality due to asthma in most developed countries (Sears and Taylor, 1994). The most obvious reason for this increase is the associated increase in asthma prevalence. However, controversy continues about the relationship between asthma therapy and mortality. The inflammatory nature of asthma is now well understood and agents which suppress the inflammatory components of asthma have been developed and are now used widely (Barnes and Pedersen, 1993). Inhaled corticosteroids have been shown to have a protective effect for both fatal and near-fatal asthma (Ernst et al, 1992). However, β_2-agonists have been incriminated as a potential contributor to asthma mortality. There has been a second and higher epidemic of asthma

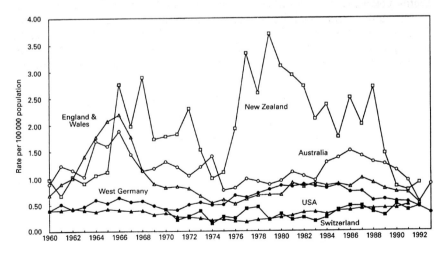

Figure 1. Trends in mortality rates for six countries (5–34 years age range). –O– Australia; –□– New Zealand; –△– England and Wales; –■– Switzerland; –▲– USA; –●– West Germany.

mortality in New Zealand in the second half of the 1970s and throughout the 1980s. This epidemic has been attributed to use of the β_2-agonist fenoterol, which was introduced into New Zealand in 1976 (Crane et al, 1989; Pearce et al, 1990; Grainger, 1991). The initial study was not well controlled for severity, but the findings were consistent with the subsequent two studies when severity had been controlled for, reporting the increased risk of death associated with fenoterol with an odds ratio of approximately 2.0.

A more recent study from the province of Saskatchewan, Canada, confirmed the high risk of death associated with the use of fenoterol (odds ratio 9.1) (Spitzer et al, 1992). However, in this study, there was also an increased risk of death associated with the use of salbutamol (odds ratio 2.8). There was also a significant correlation between an increase in the number of salbutamol canisters used per month and the risk of death. For those subjects using more than two canisters of salbutamol per month, the odds ratio increased to 29.4. While this dose-response relationship may imply causality, there was no control for severity of underlying asthma, and one might assume that the higher consumption of β_2-agonist was a marker for unstable asthma, not well managed with appropriate prophylactic therapy, which is the risk factor for death.

There is now good evidence associating β-agonist use with two epidemics of asthma deaths in the past 30 years which, together with the association of frequent β_2-agonist use and increased mortality, suggest that increased sales of β_2-agonists may be contributing to the rise in asthma mortality.

Patterns

From the few studies describing the circumstances surrounding deaths due to asthma in children, two clear patterns emerge. The first is the more traditional concept of a progressive deterioration during an acute attack, usually in a child with a background of severe persistent asthma. The second pattern is that of a sudden onset of severe airways obstruction which rapidly progresses to collapse within minutes, often without sufficient time for intervention with effective treatment. In a 3 year study of all childhood asthma deaths in the state of Victoria, this pattern was seen in 63% and was more common in those children with a prior history of mild asthma (Robertson et al, 1992b). As a result, almost all the deaths occurred outside hospital. This is in keeping with the New Zealand study (Sears et al, 1986c), where it appears that if an acute care facility is reached, the patient with severe asthma usually survives, but is in contrast to data from the United States which suggests that almost half of asthma deaths occur in hospital (Sly, 1988).

The concept of sudden death due to asthma has been increasingly recognized. In those who have died suddenly, post-mortem examination has shown a range of pathological changes ranging from the classical pattern of mucus plugging, mucosal oedema, inflammatory cell infiltrate and marked smooth muscle hypertrophy to airways that have the basic pathological changes to asthma but are empty of mucus (Reid, 1987). Recently, detailed pathological examination of patients who died from sudden-onset asthma has shown the range of histopathological features mentioned above but demonstrated a different pattern of inflammatory cell infiltrate (Sur et al, 1993). In so-called slow-onset fatal asthma, the airway inflammation is dominated by eosinophils, plasma cells and lymphocytes. In the cases of sudden-onset fatal asthma, there were fewer eosinophils and an excess of neutrophils in the airway mucosa. These differences suggest that the mechanism of inflammation and airway closure in sudden-onset fatal asthma may be quite distinct from the slow-onset fatal asthma.

A recent study from Japan has shown that patients who have survived a near-fatal episode, have reduced ventilatory response and lower airway occlusion pressure to progressive hypoxia when compared to normal subjects and to a group of subjects with asthma without a history of near-fatal episode. There was also a blunted perception of dyspnoea in this group, suggesting that a reduced central response to hypoxia may predispose patients to fatal asthma attacks (Kikuchi et al, 1994). Other authors have also reported poor perception of airway obstruction in patients with asthma (Rubinfeld and Pain, 1976; Barnes, 1992).

It is difficult to explain the circumstances of death in these patients with sudden-onset fatal asthma. It is probable that they developed a severe episode of airway obstruction which produced hypoxia. Myocardial abnormalities unrelated to treatment, in the form of contraction bands, have been reported in children dying of asthma (Drislane et al, 1987). Perhaps these children dying with apparently minor asthma have severe episodes of hypoxia and their associated myocardial abnormalities result in a fatal cardiac arrhythmia. Alternatively those children with sudden-onset fatal asthma who had the typical post-mortem findings may have had chronic airways obstruction which had not been previously recognized by themselves, their parents or their physicians.

Risk factors

A major risk factor for asthma is age. The mortality rate for asthma increases with age throughout childhood. When averaged over a 5 year period (1986–1990) in Australia, the annual rate per 100 000 population for children 0–4 years old was 0.18, for those aged 5–9 years was 0.39, 10–14 years 1.00 and for those 15–19 years 1.74, respectively, where the rate for the total population was 5.1 per 100 000. Similar trends with age are seen in other countries. Most deaths occur in the second decade, with very few under the age of 5 years. Assuming the prevalence of asthma to be approximately 20%, the annual risk of death for a child with asthma in Australia is:

1 per 100 000 asthmatics under the age of 5 years;
1 per 65 000 asthmatics between the ages of 5 and 9 years;
1 per 20 000 asthmatics between the ages of 10 and 14 years;
1 per 13 000 asthmatics between the ages of 15 and 19 years.

Most reviews of asthma mortality in children have been descriptive, with few retrospective case-control studies. In the Victorian study, following a

review of reported symptoms of previous asthma, exercise capacity, medication requirements and previous acute attacks, 33% were judged to have
had a history of mild asthma, 31% moderately severe and 36% to have had
severe asthma (Robertson et al, 1992b). A total of 22% were reported to be
symptom free in the 3 months prior to their death. Although 68% had been
hospitalized at some stage in their life, only 44% had a hospital admission
in the 12 months prior to their death. In fact, in two-thirds of deaths the parents reported that their child's asthma was either stable or improving over
the 12 months prior to death.

Other studies have proposed a profile of patients at risk of dying from
asthma (Carswell, 1985; Newcomb and Akter, 1985; Rea et al, 1986; Miller
and Strunk, 1989). This profile includes such characteristics as: chronic
severe asthma, recent hospitalization for asthma, prior life-threatening
attack, poor compliance and psychosocial disturbance. In those who have
had an episode of respiratory failure due to asthma, there is a much higher
risk of a subsequent fatal attack. When followed over a 5 year period, the
risk has been reported as 7% compared to 0.07% in those attending the
same hospital clinic who had had no episode of near-fatal asthma
(Newcomb and Akter, 1985). The risk associated with excessive β_2-agonist
use has been discussed above. The Victorian experience suggests that while
those with the above characteristics may be at increased risk, the majority
of deaths occur in children without identifiable risk factors.

Preventable factors

In the majority of descriptive studies of asthma mortality, there are four
common preventable factors which can be identified in approximately two-
thirds of the patients. These factors include: inadequate assessment and
prescribed therapy of previous asthma; poor compliance with seemingly
appropriate prescribed therapy; inadequate recognition of severity of acute
attack; delay in seeking appropriate professional help. The inadequate
assessment of previous asthma may be on the part of the patient who fails
to recognize the severity of their underlying asthma and therefore fails to
attend for a physician assessment, thereby precluding appropriate therapy.
It may also be on the part of the physician who fails to make an accurate
assessment of severity, by inadequate history, examination or failure to
make objective measurements of lung function. A physician may also fail
to prescribe an appropriate level of therapy or may prescribe inappropriate
delivery devices, reducing efficiency of the prescribed medication. Poor
compliance with prescribed therapy is a major problem in the management
of asthma resulting in widespread significant disability, in addition to mortality. In the majority of children who die from an episode with sudden
onset, it is their first severe attack. In addition to the poor perception
referred to above, patients often have no experience by which to judge the
severity at the onset of the fatal attack. There are three key factors that contribute to a delay in seeking appropriate professional help in an acute attack
of asthma: inadequate recognition of the severity; inadequate knowledge of
what action to take; denial of the severity of that attack.

If we are to reduce mortality due to asthma, we must identify environmental factors that may reduce the prevalence and severity of asthma and ensure that patients with asthma understand the need for treatment and its benefits, that they have a clear plan of how to recognize and manage a severe acute attack and that physicians are adequately trained to provide appropriate management.

PREVALENCE OF WHEEZE IN DEVELOPING COUNTRIES: IS IT CHANGING WITH DEVELOPMENT?

The true prevalence of asthma in developing countries is virtually unknown. While there have been numerous reports on the prevalence of asthma in children from developed, or more industrialized countries, the published information regarding the prevalence of asthma and risk factors in Latin American, Asian and African children is relatively small. The reported prevalence of asthma in Latin American children varies from 4.6 to 33% (Valenzuela et al, 1981; Bustos and Weller, 1982; Cruz et al, 1985; Gonzalez, 1985; Filho et al, 1986; Carrasco, 1987; Perdomo et al, 1989; Isturiz et al, 1990; Valdes et al, 1990; Arancibia et al, 1991; Mallol and Cortes, 1992; Oyarzun et al, 1993). However, there are wide variations in methodology between those studies with differing definitions, questions, and study design. Therefore, much of the information may not reflect the actual prevalence of the disease. Thus the existence of true variations in the prevalence of asthma in children from different countries or communities in Latin America and other developing regions, remains very uncertain.

Most instruments used to determine the prevalence of asthma have relied on questionnaires inquiring about a history of respiratory symptoms or a doctor diagnosis of asthma. While the validity of these instruments has been demonstrated in developed countries, where chronic suppurative lung disease is uncommon, such validity may not be generalizable to the developing regions where both acute and chronic respiratory infection is a major problem. Tests of bronchial responsiveness and skin prick tests for atopy have been helpful in distinguishing symptoms likely to be due to asthma from those due to respiratory infections (Flynn, 1994), but have rarely been used in developing countries.

Recently, the prevalence of asthma in children from Australia, Chile and Switzerland was compared using the same instrument (Robertson et al, 1993). It was shown that the current prevalence of wheezing in children aged 12 years was similar in children from Australia (20.9%) and Chile (21.1%) but significantly lower in Switzerland (6.0%); for 7-year-olds it was 23.1% in Australia, 26.5% in Chile and 7.4% in Switzerland, suggesting that the genetic, educational and environmental factors, among others, might be responsible for regional differences in asthma prevalence.

Using the same methodology, the prevalence of current asthma in school children living in localities with a high degree of air pollution has been shown to be significantly lower (range 17–18%) than those living in cities with no evident air pollution (range 26–27%) (Mallol et al; unpublished data). This paradoxical observation of lower or equal prevalence of asthma in children living in areas with high air pollution has also been found when assessing bronchial responsiveness to methacholine in schoolchildren from two Chilean cities, Santiago (polluted air) and Los Andes (nonpolluted air): the difference in the prevalence of bronchial hyperresponsiveness was not statistically significant (Oyarzun et al, 1993). A very similar observation has been reported for German children from two cities with different levels of air pollution (von Mutius et al, 1994a). The reasons for this paradox are unclear, but von Mutius has suggested it may relate to frequent infections in infancy associated with increased family size (von Mutius et al, 1994b).

The relationship between transiently high levels of atmospheric pollution and acute presentation with respiratory symptoms is well known. There is one study from Cuba relating acute respiratory diseases and acute bronchial asthma in children with air pollution and air temperature (Molina et al, 1989). The authors found that there was an increased number of asthma consultations on days with higher levels of air pollution and they also reported higher rates of acute respiratory infections associated with periods of lower air temperature. In another study, from Rio de Janeiro, Brazil (Penna and Duchiade, 1991), a direct relationship was suggested between air pollution and infantile mortality due to pneumonia. Unfortunately, no information regarding asthma is provided by the authors. In a recent survey undertaken in 1994 that included 4400 children aged 7 years and 4200 aged 13 years from Santiago, Chile, a city with a high rate of air pollution, it was found that the prevalence of asthma in the last 12 months for children aged 7 and 13 years was 17% and 11%, respectively (Mallol et al; unpublished data).

The risk factors for asthma in children from the developing regions also vary from one country to another depending on climate, socio-economic conditions, race, and cultural background. Risk factors for asthma in developing countries include: crowded houses, tobacco smoke, use of kerosene or wood stoves, use of a fan whilst sleeping, living in coastal and humid areas, helminthic infection, sudden temperature change, weather changes, smog, viral respiratory infections, and a family history of asthma (Molina et al, 1989; Perdomo et al, 1989; Isturiz et al, 1990; Valdes et al, 1990; Arancibia et al, 1991; Robertson et al, 1993). However, the impact of each of these risk factors in determining the prevalence of asthma in children from different communities is unknown. There is some information on the prevalence of asthma in schoolchildren from Brazil (Filho et al, 1986; Rosario et al, 1986; Fritscher et al, 1994) indicating the prevalence of asthma ranging from 4.5 to 19%. Unfortunately, most of these studies have methodological problems and should be interpreted carefully.

The figures for the prevalence of asthma in children from Asia and Africa are considerably lower than that reported from other industrialized countries. In China the figures reported ranged from 1 to 2.4% (Zhong et al, 1990; National Cooperative Pediatric Group, 1993). In a recent study of Chinese children while the prevalence of recent wheeze was only 1.1%, the prevalence of other atopy was high: history of eczema, 10.4%; positive skin prick tests, 40% (Leung and Jenkins, 1994). In Hong Kong and Taiwan, the prevalence of asthma in children has been reported to be 15 and 6% respectively (Hsieh and Shen, 1988; Leung et al, 1994a). Using the same methodology, Keeley and Neil (1991), in Zimbabwe, found significant differences in the prevalence of reversible airways obstruction between children living in two rural regions (0.1 and 3.1%) and one urban (5.8%) region (Keeley et al, 1991). A similar survey of the Xhosa children in South Africa showed the prevalence of asthma to be 3.2% in the urban group and 0.1% in the rural group (Van Niekerk et al, 1979).

It seems that there are true differences in asthma prevalence in children living in different regions of the world that cannot be explained just by the level of development or race nor by methodological aspects. The reasons why the prevalence changes from one locality to another are in fact unknown. However, it is most probable that the degree of education, the environmental control, diet, the access to high quality health care, genetics and other reasons would explain such regional differences in the prevalence of respiratory symptoms suggestive of asthma in children.

In relatively isolated localities with low level of industrialization the prevalence has been reported to be as high as that from industrialized cities with higher migration rates. One possible explanation could be the larger expected rate of consanguinity. In Isla de Coche, a Venezuelan island in the Caribbean, where consanguinity is common, the prevalence of asthma in children is reported to be 42% (Palenque et al, personal communication). The impact of environment has been demonstrated in several studies of migration of racial groups where migration occurs from a region of low prevalence of asthma to a region of high prevalence. The migrants acquire the high prevalence of asthma in their new region (Waite et al, 1980; Leung et al, 1994a).

In the near future, many of the questions regarding the prevalence of asthma in children from developing countries will be answered by international studies of asthma and allergies using the same methodology combining history with measurements of bronchial responsiveness. Such a major study will hopefully provide information on risk factors for asthma, the spectrum of morbidity and mortality.

At present, there is surprisingly little information published regarding the prevalence of asthma, and morbidity and mortality due to asthma in children from developing regions of the world. In countries where the prevalence is so low and the significance of the competing illnesses so high, data collection about asthma has not received a high priority and is consequently scanty and unreliable. The data that are available would suggest that morbidity, reflected by hospital admission rates and the mortality rates due to asthma are extremely low or negligible in developing countries. As attention to asthma increases in these regions, patterns of morbidity will be more clearly defined with the consequent requirement for treatment. Effective treatment for asthma is relatively expensive and to a certain extent is a luxury of the wealthy countries. In the United States, the annual expenditure on asthma has been estimated at 6.2 billion dollars in 1990 (Weiss et al,

1992). Clearly there is a wide range of competing illnesses such as pneumonia, diarrhoea and malnutrition which would have a far higher priority for the limited health dollar available in developing countries. In developing countries, the prevalence of asthma is higher in the urban than rural population and it is interesting to speculate on the impact increasing urbanization will have on the prevalence of asthma.

Asthma has been given a great deal of attention over recent years in the developed countries, where it makes a significant contribution to morbidity and mortality in childhood. However, the paucity of attention given to asthma in developing countries to date is a reflection of its relative lack of importance amongst a range of competing health problems, such as adequate nutrition, immunization and early recognition and treatment of infections.

SUMMARY

The prevalence of asthma varies throughout the world. Factors which contribute to the variation include: the use of different definitions of asthma for epidemiological studies, language and cultural factors, genetic and environmental factors. Environmental factors which have been widely studied include: components of air pollution, maternal smoking, allergen load and diet. In several countries, where serial measurements have been made, there has been a consistent rise in the prevalence of asthma. While most studies have reported an increase based on the responses to questionnaires, the increase has been supported by an increase in objective measures of bronchial hyperresponsiveness and an increase in hospital admission rates for asthma.

There is a similar variation in mortality rate for asthma between countries. While linked to prevalence rates, the variation in mortality rates is not adequately explained by them. Risk factors include: excessive use of β_2 agonists, age, chronic severe asthma, repeated hospitalizations for asthma, poor compliance and psychosocial disturbance.

In developing countries, the true prevalence of asthma is virtually unkwown, due to both methodological problems and competing health issues. It can also be difficult to distinguish symptoms of asthma from those of chronic suppurative lung disease. In general, the reported prevalence rates of asthma from developing countries are considerably lower than from other more industrialized countries.

REFERENCES

Anderson HR, Bailey PA, Cooper JS et al (1983) Medical care of asthma and wheezing in illness in children: a community survey. *Journal of Epidemiology and Community Health* **37:** 180–186.
Anderson HR, Bland JM, Patel S & Peckham C (1986) The natural history of asthma in childhood. *Journal of Epidemiology and Community Health* **40:** 121–129.
Anderson HR, Butland BK & Strachan DP (1994) Trends in prevalence and severity of childhood asthma. *British Medical Journal* **308:** 1600–1604.

Anto JM, Sun J, Rodrigueuz-Roisin R et al (1989) Community outbreaks of asthma associated with inhalation of soybean dust. *New England Journal of Medicine* **320**: 1097–1102.

Arancibia L, Pernas M, Almiral J & Bacallao J (1991) Determination of peak expiratory flow in asthmatic children between crisis. *Revista Cubana Investigaciones Biomedicas* **10**: 49–55.

Arm JP, Horton CE, Supr BW et al (1989) The effects of dietary supplementation with fish oil lipids on the airways response in inhaled allergen in bronchial asthma. *American Review of Respiratory Disease* **139**: 1395–1400.

Asher MI, Pattemore, PK, Harrison AC et al (1988) International comparison of the prevalence of bronchial hyperresponsiveness and asthma symptoms. *American Review of Respiratory Disease* **138**: 524–529.

Barnes PJ (1992) Poorly perceived asthma. *Thorax* **47**: 408–409.

Barnes PJ & Pedersen S (1993) Efficacy and safety of inhaled corticosteriods in asthma. *American Review of Respiratory Disease* **148**: S1–S26.

Bauman A (1993) Has the prevalence of asthma symptoms increased in Australian children. *Journal of Paediatrics and Child Health* **29**: 424–428.

Braback L, Breborowicz A, Dreborg S et al (1994) Atopic sensitisation and respiratory symptoms among Polish and Swedish school children. *Clinical and Experimental Allergy* **24**: 826–835.

British Thoracic Society Research Committee (1984) Accuracy of death certificates in bronchial asthma: accuracy of certification procedures during the confidential inquiry by the British Thoracic Society. *Thorax* **38**: 505–509.

Burney PGJ (1985) A diet rich in sodium may potentiate asthma: epidemiological evidence for a new hypothesis. In Holland WW (ed.) *Proceedings of Fogarty International Centre Workshop on Aetiology of Asthma*. National Institutes of Health, 25–27 June 1985.

Burney PGJ (1989) The effect of death certification practice on recorded national asthma mortality rates. *Review of Epidemiology, Sante Publique* **37**: 385–389.

Burney PGJ, Chinn S & Rona RJ (1990) Has the prevalence of asthma increased in children? Evidence from the national study of health and growth 1973–86. *British Medical Journal* **300**: 1306–1310.

Burney PGJ, Britton JR, Chinn S et al (1986). Response to inhaled histamine and 24 hour sodium excretion. *British Medical Journal* **292**: 1483–1486.

Burr ML, Butland BK, King S & Vaughan-Williams E (1989) Changes in asthma prevalence: two surveys 15 years apart. *Archives of Disease in Childhood* **64**: 1452–1456.

Bustos G & Weller J (1982) Asma en el nino: consideraciones acerca de su verdadera prevalencia. *Archivos Argentinos de Pediatria* **80**: 203–212.

Carmen PG & Landau LI (1990) Increased paediatric admissions with asthma in Western Australia—a problem of diagnosis? *The Medical Journal of Australia* **152**: 123–126.

Carr W, Zeitel L & Weiss K (1992) Variations in asthma hospitalisations and deaths in New York city. *American Journal of Public Health* **82**: 59–65.

Carrasco E (1987) Epidemiology of asthma in Latin American children. *Chest* **91**: 935–975.

Carswell F (1985) Thirty deaths from asthma. *Archives of Disease in Childhood* **60**: 25–28.

Clifford RD, Pugsley A, Radford M & Holgate ST (1987) Symptoms, atopy, and bronchial response to methacholine in parents with asthma and their children. *Archives of Disease in Childhood* **62**: 66–73.

Crane J, Pearce N, Flatt A et al (1989) Prescribed fenoterol and death from asthma in New Zealand, 1981–83: case-control study. *Lancet* **i**: 918–922.

Cruz E, Marquez R & Ortiz M (1985) Prevalencia del asma en escolares de 6–14 anos en Santo Domingo. *Archivos Dominicanos de Pediatria* **21**: 9–14.

Drislane FW, Samuels MA, Kozakewich H et al (1987) Myocardial contraction band lesions in patients with fatal asthma: Possible neurocardiologic mechanisms. *American Review of Respiratory Disease* **135**: 498–501.

Duffy DL, Martin NG, Battistutta D et al (1990) Genetics of asthma and hayfever in Australian twins. *American Review of Respiratory Disease* **142**: 1351–1358.

Edfors-Lubs ML (1971) Allergy in 7000 twin pairs. *Acta Allergologica* **26**: 249–285.

Ernst P, Spitzer WO, Suissa S et al (1992) Risk of fatal and near-fatal asthma in relation to inhaled corticosteriod use. *Journal of the American Medical Association* **268**: 3462–3464.

Evans D, Levison MJ, Feldman CH et al (1987) The impact of passive smoking on emergency room visits of urban children with asthma. *American Review of Respiratory Disease* **135**: 567–572.

Filho R, Augusto N, Eldecastro S & Gutierrez M (1986) Prevalencia de asma bronquica em consultas peditricas. *Revista Medica deParana* **44**: 57–59.

Fitzgerald JM, Sears MR & Roberts RS (1988) Symptoms of asthma and airway hyperresponsiveness to methacholine in a population of Canadian schoolchildren. *American Review of Respiratory Disease* 137: 285.

Flynn MG (1994) Respiratory symptoms, bronchial responsiveness and atopy in Fijian and Indian children. *American Journal of Respiratory and Critical Care Medicine* 150: 415–420.

Frischer T, Studnicka M, Neumann M & Geotz M (1992) Determinants of airway response to challenge with distilled water in a population sample of children aged 7 to 10 years old. *Chest* 102: 764–770.

Fritscher CC, Severo RD, Fagondes GS et al (1994) Modificacoes na prevalencia de asma bronquica em escolares de Portp Alegre. *Jornal Brasilerio de Pneumologia* 20: 6–10.

Gergen PJ, Mullally DI & Evans R (1988) National survey of prevalence of asthma among children in the United States, 1976 to 1980. *Pediatrics* 81: 1–7.

Gleibermann L (1973) Blood pressure and dietary salt in human populations. *Ecology of Food and Nutrition* 2: 143–156.

Gonzalez M (1985) Prevalencia del asma bronquial en escolares de 6–14 anos en Santo Domingo, Republica Dominicana. *Archivos Dominicanos de Pediatria* 21: 9–14.

Grainger J, Woodman K, Pearce N et al (1991) Prescribed fenoterol and death from asthma in New Zealand, 1981–87: a further case-control study. *Thorax* 46: 105–111.

Haby MM, Anderson SD & Peat JK (1994) An exercise challenge protocol for epidemiological studies of asthma in children: comparison with histamine challenge. *European Respiratory Journal* 1: 43–49.

Hanrahan J, Tager I, Segal M et al (1992) Effect of prenatal smoking on infant lung function. *American Review of Respiratory Disease* 145: 1129–1135.

Hsieh KH & Shen JJ (1988) Prevalence of childhood asthma in Taipei, Taiwan, and other Asian Pacific countries. *Journal of Asthma* 25: 73–82.

Holt PG, McMenamin C & Nelson D (1990) Primary sensitisation to inhalant allergens during infancy. *Pediatric Allergy and Immunology* 1: 3–13.

Inman WHW & Adelstein AM (1969) Rise and fall of asthma mortality in England and Wales in relation to use of pressurised aerosols. *Lancet* ii: 279–285.

ISAAC—International Study of Asthma and Allergies in Childhood Manual (1992).

Isturiz G, Rosquete R, Armegol R et al (1990) Variability in asthma prevalance in a tropical country. *Gaceta Medica de Caracas* 98: 182–187.

Javid A, Cushley MJ & Bone MF (1988) Effect of dietary salt on bronchial reactivity to histamine in asthma. *British Medical Journal* 297: 454.

Jenkins MA, Rubinfeld AR, Robertson CF & Bowes G (1992) Accuracy of asthma death statistics in Australia. *Australian Journal of Public Health* 16: 427–429.

Jenkins M, Hopper J, Bowes G et al (1994) Adult asthma: What are the childhood risk factors and has it increased over the last generation. *American Journal of Respiratory and Critical Care Medicine* 149: A574.

Kikuchi Y, Okabe S, Tamura G et al (1994) Chemosensitivity and perception of dyspnoea in patients with a history of near-fatal asthma. *New England Journal of Medicine* 330: 1329–1334.

Keeley DJ, Neil P & Gallivan S (1991) Comparison of the prevalence of reversible airways obstruction in rural and urban Zimbabwean children. *Thorax* 46: 549–553.

Kuhni CE & Sennhauser FH (1995) The Yentl syndrome in childhood asthma: risk factors for undertreatment in Swiss children. *Pediatric Pulmonology* 19: 156–160.

Kun HY, Oates RK & Mellis CM (1993) Hospital admissions and attendances for asthma—a true increase? *The Medical Journal of Australia* 159: 312–313.

Lang DM & Polansky M (1994) Patterns of asthma mortality in Philadelphia from 1969 to 1991. *New England Journal of Medicine* 331: 1542–1546.

Leung R & Jenkins M (1994) Asthma, allergy and atopy in southern Chinese school students. *Clinical and Experimenal Allergy* 24: 353–358.

Leung R, Bishop J & Robertson (1994a) Prevalence of wheeze in Hong Kong schoolchildren—An international comparison. *European Respiratory Journal* 7: 2046–2049.

Leung RC, Carlin JB, Burdon JGW & Czarny D (1994b) Asthma, allergy and atopy in Asian immigrants in Melbourne. *The Medical Journal of Australia* 161: 418–425.

Mallol J & Cortes F (1992) Prevalence of asthma in Chilean school children. *American Review of Respiratory Disease* 145: A662.

Manfreda J, Becker A, Wang P et al (1993) Trends in physician diagnosed asthma prevalence in Manitoba between 1980 and 1990. *Chest* 103: 151–157.

Miller BD & Strunk RC (1989) Circumstances surrounding the deaths of children due to asthma. *American Journal of Disease of Children* **143:** 1294–1299.

Mitchell EA (1985) International trends in hospital admission rates for asthma. *Archives of Disease in Childhood* **60:** 376–378.

Mitchell EA & Asher MI (1994) Prevalence, severity and medical management of asthma in European school children in 1895 and 1991. *Journal of Paediatrics and Child Health* **30:** 398–402.

Mitchell EA, Anderson HR, Freeling P & White PT (1990) Why are hospital admission and mortality rates for childhood asthma higher in New Zealand than in the United Kingdom? *Thorax* **45:** 176–182.

Molina E, Barcelo C & Ceballos R (1989) Contaminantes primarios de la atmosfera, temperatura del aire, enfermedad respiratoria aguda y asma bronquial en ninos. *Revista Cubana de Pediatria* **61:** 215–227.

National Cooperative Pediatric Group on Asthma Research P. R. China, Beijing 100020 (1993) A national survey on the prevalence of asthma among 0–14 year old population in China (1988–1990). *Chinese Journal of Tuberculosis and Respiratory Diseases* **16:** 83.

Neas LM, Dockery DW, Ware JH et al (1991) Association of indoor nitrogen dioxide with respiratory symptoms and pulmonary function in children. *American Journal of Epidemiology* **134:** 204–219.

Newcomb RW & Akter J (1985) Respiratory failure from asthma. A marker for children with high morbidity and mortality. *American Journal of Disease of Children* **142:** 1401–1404.

Nicolai T, Mutius EV, Reitmeir P & Wist M (1993) Reactivity to cold air hyperventilation in normal and in asthmatic children in a survey of 5,697 schoolchildren in Southern Bavaria. *American Review of Respiratory Disease* **147:** 565–572.

Ninan TK & Russell G (1992) *British Medical Journal* **304:** 873–875.

Oshima Y, Ishizaki T, Miyamoto T et al (1964) A study of Tokyo-Yokohama asthma among Japanese. *American Review of Respiratory Disease* **90:** 632–634.

Oyarzun M, Pino P, Ancic P et al (1993) Bronchial hyperresponsiveness and air pollution: the baseline of a cohort study in Chilean school children. *American Review of Respiratory Disease* **147:** A826.

Pearce N, Grainger J, Aitkinson M et al (1990) Case-control study of prescribed fenoterol and death from asthma in New Zealand, 1977–81. *Thorax* **45:** 170–175.

Peat JK, Salome CM, Sedgwick CS et al (1988) A prospective study of bronchial hyperresponsiveness and respiratory symptoms in a population of Australian schoolchildren. *Clinical and Experimenal Allergy* **19:** 299–306.

Peat JK, Salome CM & Woolcock AJ (1992a) Factors associated with bronchial hyperresponsiveness in Australian adults and children. *European Respiratory Journal* **5:** 921–929.

Peat JK, Haby M, Spijker J et al (1992b) Prevalence of asthma in adult in Busselton, Western Australia. *British Medical Journal* **305:** 1326–1329.

Peat JK, Tovey E, Mellis CM et al (1993) Importance of house dust mite and Alternaria allergens in childhood asthma: an epidemiological study in two climatic regions of Australia. *Clinical and Experimental Allergy* **23:** 812–820.

Peat JK, van den Berg RH, Green WF et al (1994) Changes in prevalence of asthma in Australian children. *British Medical Journal* **308:** 1591–1596.

Penna ML & Duchiade M (1991) Contaminacion del aire y mortalidad infantile por neumonia. *Boleti de la Ofina Panamericana de Salud* **110:** 199–206.

Perdomo D, Benarroch L, Marcano W et al (1989) Allergy and parasites: an association dissoluble. *Immunologia Clinica* **89:** 223–226.

Pope CA & Dockery DW (1992) Acute health effects of PM_{10} pollution on symptomatic and asymptomatic children. *American Review of Respiratory Disease* **145:** 1123–1128.

Rea HH, Scragg R, Jackson et al (1986) A case control study of deaths from asthma. *Thorax* **41:** 833–839.

Reid LM (1987) The presence or absence of bronchial mucus in fatal asthma. *Journal of Clinical Immunology* **148:** 713–719.

Riedler J, Reade T, Dalton M et al (1995) Hypertonic saline challenge in an epidemiological survey of asthma in children. *American Journal of Critical Care and Respiratory Medicine* **150:** 1632–1639.

Robertson CF, Heycock E, Bishop J et al (1991) Prevalence of asthma in Melbourne schoolchildren: Changes over 26 years. *British Medical Journal* **302:** 1116–1118.

Robertson CF, Bishop J, Dalton M et al (1992a) Prevalence of asthma in regional Victorian school-children. *The Medical Journal of Australia* **156:** 831–833.

Robertson CF, Rubinfeld AR & Bowes G (1992b) Pediatric asthma deaths in Victoria: the mild are at risk. *Pediatric Pulmonology* **13:** 95–100.

Robertson CF, Bishop J, Sennhauser FH et al (1993) International comparison of asthma prevalence in children: Australia, Switzerland and Chile. *Pediatric Pulmonology* **16:** 219–226.

Rosario NA, Sevilla E & Branco ME (1986) Prevalencia de Asma Broquica em Consulta Pediatrica. *Revista Medica de Parana* **44:** 57–59.

Rubinfeld AR & Pain MC (1976) Perception of asthma. *Lancet* **i:** 882–884.

Scadding JG (1963) Meaning of diagnostic terms in bronchopulmonary disease. *British Medical Journal* **2:** 1425–1430.

Schwartz J, Gold D, Dockery DW et al (1990) Predictors of asthma and persistent wheeze in a national sample of children in the United States. *American Review of Respiratory Disease* **142:** 555–562.

Sears MR & Taylor DR (1994) The β_2-agonist controversy: Observations, explanations and relationship to asthma epidemiology. *Drug Safety* **11:** 259–283.

Sears MR, Rea HH, Beaglehole R et al (1985) Asthma mortality in New Zealand: a two year national study. *New Zealand Medical Journal* **98:** 271–275.

Sears MR, Jones DT, Holloway et al (1986a) Prevalence of bronchial reactivity to inhaled methacholine in New Zealand children. *Thorax* **41:** 283–289.

Sears M, Rea HH, Fenwick J et al (1986c) Deaths from asthma in New Zealand. *Archives of Disease in Childhood* **61:** 6–10.

Sears MR, Rea HH, DeBoer G et al (1986b). Accuracy of certification of deaths due to asthma: a national study. *American Journal of Epidemiology* **124:** 1004–1011.

Seaton A, Godden DJ & Brown K (1994) Increase in asthma: a more toxic environment or more susceptible population? *Thorax* **49:** 171–174.

Sharpin D, Birnbaum J, Haddi E et al (1991) Altitude and allergy to housedust mites. *American Review of Respiratory Disease* **143:** 983–986.

Sly RM (1988) Mortality from asthma. *Journal of Allergy and Clinical Immunology* **82:** 705–717.

Speight ANP, Lee DA & Hey EN (1983) Underdiagnosis and undertreatment of asthma in childhood. *British Medical Journal* **286:** 1253–1255.

Speizer FE, Doll R & Heaf P (1968) Observations on recent increase in mortality from asthma. *British Medical Journal* **1:** 335–339.

Spitzer WO, Suissa S, Ernst P et al (1992) The use of β_2-agonists and the risk of death and near death from asthma. *New England Journal of Medicine* **326:** 501–506.

Sporik R, Holgate S, Platts-Mills T & Cogswell J (1990) Exposure to house dust mite allergen (Der p1) and the development of asthma in childhood. *New England Journal of Medicine* **323:** 502–507.

Strachan DP & Anderson HR (1992) Trends in hospital admission rates for asthma in children. *British Medical Journal* **304:** 819–820.

Strachan DP, Anderson HR, Limb ES et al (1994) A national survey of asthma prevalence, severity and treatment in Great Britain. *Archives of Disease in Childhood* **70:** 174–178.

Sur S, Crotty TB, Kephart GM et al (1993) Sudden-onset fatal asthma. A distinct entity with few eosinophils and relatively more neutrophils in the airways submucosa? *American Review of Respiratory Disease* **148:** 713–719.

Taylor B, Wadsworth J, Golding J & Butler N (1983) Breast feeding, eczema and hayfever. *Journal of Epidemiology and Community Health* **37:** 95–99.

Toelle BG, Peat JK, Salome CM et al (1992) Towards a definition of asthma for epidemiology. *American Review of Respiratory Disease* **146:** 633–637.

US Environmental Protection Agency (1992) Respiratory health of passive smoking: Lung cancer and other disorders EPA/600/6–90/006F. Washington, DC: US EPA.

Valdes J, Herrera, Riambou J & Otero R (1990) Bronchial asthma in children; social and environmental factors that influence it. *Revista Cubana de Pediatria* **62:** 365–375.

Valenzuela P, Gomez G & Galleguillos F (1981) Prevalencia del asma bronquial en escolares de Santiago. *Revista Medica de Chile* **109:** 259–266.

Van Niekerk CH, Weinberg SC, Shore SC et al (1979) Prevalence of asthma: a comparative study of urban and rural Xhosa children. *Clinical Allergy* **9:** 319–324.

Von Mutius E, Martinez FD, Fritzsch C et al (1994a) Prevalence of asthma and atopy in two areas of West and East Germany. *American Journal of Respiratory and Critical Care Medicine* **149:** 358–364.

Von Mutius, Martinez FD, Fitzsch C et al (1994b) Skin test reactivity and number of siblings. *British Medical Journal* **308**: 692–695.

Waite DA, Eyles EF, Tonkin SL & O'Donnell TV (1980) Asthma prevalence in Tokelauan children in two environments. *Clinical Allergy* **10**: 71–75.

Weiss KB & Wagener DK (1990) Changing patterns of asthma mortality. Identifying target populations at high risk. *Journal of the American Medical Association* **264**: 1683–1687.

Weiss KB, Gergen PJ & Hodgson TA (1992) An economic evaluation of asthma in the United States. *New England Journal of Medicine* **326**: 862–866.

Whincup PH, Cook DG, Strachan DP & Papacosta O (1993) Time trends in respiratory symptoms in childhood over a 24 year period. *Archives of Disease in Childhood* **68**: 729–734.

Wright A, Holberg C, Martinez F et al (1991) Relationship of parental smoking to wheezing and non-wheezing lower respiratory tract illnesses in infancy. *Journal of Pediatrics* **118**: 207–214.

Young SA, Le Souef PN, Geelhoed G et al (1991) The influence of family history of asthma and parental smoking on the level of airway responsiveness in infancy. *New England Journal of Medicine* **324**: 1168–1173.

Zhong NS, Chen RC, Yang MO et al (1990) Bronchial hyperresponsiveness in young students of southern China: relation to respiratory symptoms diagnosed asthma, and risk factors. *Thorax* **45**: 860–865.

3

Airway inflammation: is it relevant to childhood asthma?

K. RAJESHWAR RAO
JOHN O. WARNER

The first information on the pathology of asthma was gained from post-mortem examination, and detailed in Osler's textbook of medicine published in 1892. He described the changes of widespread mucosal plugging of the airways resulting in air trapping and hyperinflated lungs. It has been confirmed that the tenacious material forming such plugs contains inflammatory cells in addition to plasma proteins and sloughed epithelial cells (Dunnill, 1960; Dunnill et al, 1969; James et al, 1989). It has also been shown that the airway wall is affected with thickening of the smooth muscle layer and sub basement-membrane fibrosis. In addition there is considerable squamous and goblet cell metaplasia (Dunnill et al, 1969; Hossain and Heard, 1970) and accumulation of inflammatory cells (Bentley et al, 1992). These changes are mirrored in the sputum from asthmatic patients, with clumps of epithelial cells, eosinophils and airway casts consisting of plasma proteins (Naylor, 1962; Dunnill, 1978; Laitenen et al, 1985). Growing evidence from bronchoscopic studies suggests that similar changes exist in the airways of even mild asthmatics (Beasley et al, 1989; Laitenen et al, 1993) though this was originally established on post-mortem studies when death was not due to asthma (Sobonya, 1984). The structural changes are consistent with chronic inflammation of a mucus secreting surface characterized by vascular dilatation, increased permeability of blood vessels, exudation of plasma and cells and by emptying of goblet cells (Florey, 1962). Epithelial shedding is probably due to damage by eosinophil cytotoxic proteins (Gleich et al, 1979), and this in turn leads to attempts at repair with the laying down of sub basement-membrane collagen (Roche et al, 1989).

In allergic asthma, allergen is phagocytosed and processed by antigen presenting cells (APCs) which are mainly dendritic cells and alveolar macrophages in the airway mucosa (Holt, 1993). APCs then migrate to regional lymph nodes in the airways where they present antigens, along with class 2 major histocompatibility complex (MHC) molecules, to lymphocytes. CD4+ T-lymphocytes, so-called helper cells, recognize the antigen molecules on the APCs and undergo sensitization such that subsequent antigen exposure leads to the production of cytokines, mainly

Baillière's Clinical Paediatrics—
Vol. 3, No. 2, May 1995
ISBN 0–7020–1986–0

277

interleukins (IL)-2, 3, 4, 5, interferon gamma (INF-γ) and granulocyte-macrophage colony stimulating factor (GM-CSF). Recent evidence has shown that increased levels of activated T-lymphocytes, of both the CD4 and CD8 type are present in the peripheral blood of children with asthma (Gemou-Engesaeth et al, 1994). In allergic individuals, there is a selective development of subsets of T-lymphocytes of the Th_2 type, producing IL-4, IL-5, IL-10 and IL-13 (rather than IL-2 and IFN-γ that come from the Th_1 cells) which is promoted in an autocrine response by IL-4 and inhibited by IL-12 (Romagnani, 1992; Scott, 1993) secreted primarily by macrophages (Figure. 1).

B-lymphocytes are activated on exposure to specific antigen and CD4+ T-cells, and release specific IgE antibodies under the influence of IL-4, IL-

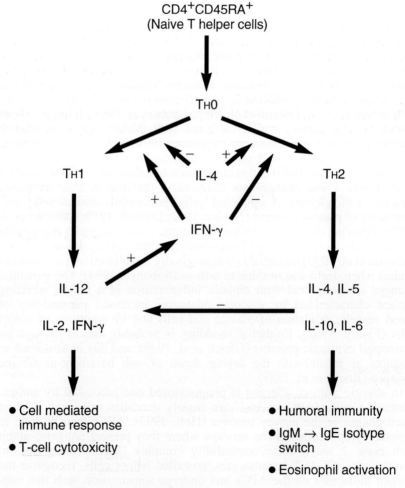

Figure 1. T-lymphocyte activation and differentiation in asthma.

13 and a combination of the CD40 molecule and its ligand. These antibodies bind to high affinity receptors on mast cells and basophils and also to low affinity receptors found on eosinophils, monocytes, lymphocytes, dendritic cells and platelets. Cross-linking of the IgE molecules by allergen on the surface of these cells leads to activation and release of a number of mediators into intercellular spaces. These include a range of preformed mediators, such as histamine, proteoglycans, proteases and heparin, but also de-novo synthesis of certain lipid-derived products. The latter are derived from two routes, the cycloxygenase pathway producing prostaglandins and thromboxanes, and the lipoxygenase pathway generating leukotrienes and hydroxy-eicosatetranoic acids (HETES). The products of mast cells mediate the immediate asthmatic response, characterized by bronchospasm, but also contribute to the development of chronic inflammation. IL-3, IL-4 and IL-10, released mainly by lymphocytes, cause further development of mast cells. The mast cell itself produces various cytokines including IL-4, to further enhance and maintain the allergic inflammatory process (Holgate et al, 1988; Bard et al, 1989; Takagi et al, 1989). IL-4 and IL-13, by producing an isotype switching (Gauchet et al, 1990), stimulate IgE secretion by B-lymphocytes (Alving et al, 1990). IgE itself causes further priming of the B-cells. Thus a cycle of self-perpetuating inflammation is established (Figure 2).

Eosinophil activation is another important process in the airway inflammation of asthma. IL-5 and to some extent GM-CSF, mainly secreted by activated CD4 T-lymphocytes, are known specifically to stimulate

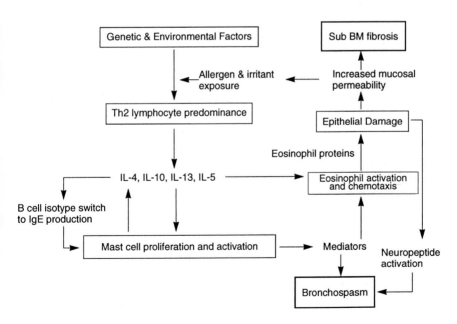

Figure 2. Pathophysiology of asthma.

eosinophil proliferation, activation and survival (Owen et al, 1987; Lopez et al, 1988; Yamaguchi et al, 1988). Often a blood and tissue eosinophilia is found in asthma (Bousquet et al, 1990), and activated eosinophils, which appear hypodense as a result of degranulation, are increased in number (Frick et al, 1989; Venge and Peterson, 1989; Adelroth et al, 1990). The activated eosinophil releases various cytotoxic proteins responsible for many of the pathological features of asthma. These include the eosinophil cationic protein (ECP), eosinophil protein-X (EPX) previously also known as eosinophil derived neurotoxin (EDN), eosinophil peroxidase (EPO), and major basic protein (MBP). These proteins reside in special cytoplasmic granules, are strongly cationic and produce significant tissue destruction. In addition, the eosinophil also secretes the lipid mediators, platelet activating factor (PAF) and the leukotriene LTC_4 (Lee et al, 1984; Shaw et al, 1984; Hallgren and Venge, 1991). Activated eosinophils are mainly responsible for the late asthmatic response by release of the various mediators mentioned above and of free oxygen radicals. These are gradually followed by other processes including the proliferation of fibroblast activity, of nerves responsible for neuropeptide release and hypertrophy and hyperplasia of the airway smooth muscle (Holgate and Church, 1993).

T-cells express other molecules on their surface, e.g. VLA-1 and VLA-2 which are called adhesion molecules. These are important for cell to cell adhesion and their increased expression, seen in asthma, suggests chronic stimulation. Another adhesion molecule, ICAM-1 (intercellular adhesion molecule), found on vascular endothelial cells, but also on upregulated bronchial epithelial cells in asthma, facilitates T-cell and eosinophil aggregation at local sites of inflammation (Diaz et al, 1989). As ICAM-1 is the molecule through which rhinovirus gains access to the cell, it is easy to hypothesize on the susceptibility of asthmatics to rhinovirus infection (Johnston et al, 1993a).

A close link exists between the mast cell, the leukocyte and sensory nerves (Nilsson et al, 1990). Mast cell histamine results in the release of neuropeptides (Substance P, Neurokinin A, CGRP, VIP) from nerves resulting in cough, sneezing and itching (Alving et al, 1990).

The functional consequences of the structural changes are a narrowing of the airways on exposure to stimuli that do not affect normal lungs. The increased responsiveness is due partly to increased permeability but also to thickening of the airway wall (Wiggs et al, 1992). Resistance tends to reach a plateau in normal airways but can reach infinity in asthma due to near-closure of the airways. The relationship between wall thickness and muscle shortening is also applicable to muscle relaxation, which accounts for the reversibility seen in asthma.

THE GENETIC BASIS FOR ASTHMA

Asthma is a result of a complex interaction between inherited and environmental factors. We now know that a number of ante- and postnatal events prime the infant's immune system which leads to the development of atopy and asthma. There is definitely a strong familial link with atopy but a precise genetic basis still eludes us. Previous studies have had totally conflicting results as to the inheritance of high IgE production, allergy and asthma (Blumenthal, 1981; Hasstedt et al, 1983; Borecki et al, 1985). It has long been known that the incidence of allergy is higher in monozygotic than in dizygotic twins (Lubs, 1972; Hanson et al, 1991) and correlates to the number of atopic relatives (Raeburn, 1990). Atopy as well as asthma has a higher incidence in boys than in girls (Sears, 1993). A study from Oxford, UK by Cookson et al (1989), evoked great interest in the association of a dominant gene on chromosome 11 with atopy. The population for this study was from a highly selective lineage, and other workers have been unable to replicate these results with a less biased selection of populations (Amelung et a!, 1992; Lympany et al, 1992; Rich et al, 1992). Recently, a significant linkage has been shown between IgE production and the cytokine gene cluster *5q31* on chromosome 5 (Marsh et al, 1994). Speculation on whether a single gene or, more likely, multiple genes are involved in atopy continues. However, such genes must have an influence on various aspects of immune responsiveness; indeed allergy may be seen as the commonest manifestation of immune deficiency (Warner and Warner, 1993).

PATHOPHARMACOLOGY OF ASTHMA

The international consensus statement in 1992 on the diagnosis and management of asthma (Sheffer, 1992) and the follow-up statement from the International Paediatric Asthma Consensus group (Warner et al, 1992) were long overdue guidelines for the management of asthma all over the world. It is the only treatable condition in the developed world that continues to increase, with reports of a doubling of prevalence in the last two to three decades (Burr et al, 1989; Shaw et al, 1990; Ninan and Russell, 1992). As our understanding of the underlying inflammatory basis for asthma has improved, the management strategies have moved away from focusing on symptomatic relief to the use of anti-inflammatory agents. At present the only two groups of drugs that have a proven role in this respect are corticosteroids and inhaled sodium cromoglycate. In standard doses, despite prolonged and energetic usage, neither has been shown to normalize lung function, bronchial hyperresponsiveness or histology (Warner, 1993b). Only the prolonged use of oral or very high dose inhaled steroids have a significant disease modifying role, but at the high cost of growth retardation and other potentially dangerous side effects in the growing child (Warner, 1993b).

Anti-inflammatory drugs given over a prolonged period of time have an important role in suppressing the processes of inflammation and thereby preventing chronic and irreversible airway changes. However, we have as yet been unable to alter the natural history of the condition despite following established protocols.

Sodium cromoglycate and nedocromil sodium

Sodium cromoglycate was introduced into asthma management as a mast cell stabilizer. It has been shown to have an important suppressive effect on the early asthmatic response, which is mainly mast cell mediated. But it also seems to play a part in suppressing the pathological changes in chronic asthma, probably by controlling the recruitment and activation of other inflammatory cells including eosinophils. Nedocromil sodium is a much more recent addition, developed to have a more active role in the suppression of the chronic inflammatory changes. It has been shown to have a 10 times greater potency of action in suppressing the activation of inflammatory cells. It also seems to inhibit platelet activation, and has an effect on neuronal reflexes. These two drugs have a place as prophylactic agents for the control of mild to moderately severe asthma as outlined in present recommendations. They are the least toxic of all anti-asthma drugs and are worthy of trial in all patients not controlled with the occasional use of a bronchodilator alone. However, a significant proportion of patients fail to respond, necessitating the use of stronger anti-inflammatory drugs, which presently means inhaled steroids.

Corticosteroids

Initially, oral steroids were found to be very useful in the management of both acute episodes and the chronic asthma state and were used regularly until the problems of side effects started becoming obvious. This led to the development of the inhaled esters of steroids which were more specific at targeting the lung and required a much lower dosage to be effective. Their efficacy is beyond doubt as witnessed by their usage for over 20 years. However, the problems of systemic absorption remain, with the potential for long-term side effects, especially in the growing child. Newer drugs are being introduced now which are reported to be more efficiently removed by first pass metabolism in the liver thus ensuring minimal systemic activity. Steroids act at multiple steps in the inflammatory pathway. They act on the T-lymphocyte reducing cytokine production, and act independently to suppress eosinophil and mast cell recruitment. They also suppress oedema by decreasing vascular permeability, and have an effect on bronchial smooth muscle. However, the potential for side effects stems from their effects on glucose, lipid and protein metabolism, as well as their tendency to suppress the hypothalamic-pituitary-adrenal axis. Thus the problems of growth suppression and osteoporosis, along with a centripetal redistribution of fat, hypertension and mood changes are all potential hurdles in the successful long-term management of the child with asthma. The lowest dose that produces a satisfactory response should, therefore, be the aim in asthma management, especially in childhood. This approach may, however, not be compatible with maximal suppression of airway inflammation. A balance between potential for side effects and efficacy dictates the current cautious therapeutic approach, but understanding of the mechanisms would suggest a more aggressive approach. Perhaps the use of the new generation of inhaled steroids will facilitate the disease modification.

Short- and long-acting β_2 sympathomimetics

It has long been known that adrenaline has bronchodilator properties, and it has been used successfully in emergency management in acute asthma and anaphylaxis. However, its effect as a cardio-stimulant has limited its usefulness, and led to the development of more selective β_2-stimulants, the vast majority of this type of receptor being in the lung. Further modifications have allowed these drugs to be used in inhaled form, reducing the dose and improving deposition. The action of these drugs is on the bronchial smooth muscle via the cyclic adenosine monophosphate (AMP) pathway. They also inhibit the activation of mast cells, thus having a potent effect on the early asthmatic reaction. They have been used previously on a regular basis for relief of symptoms, but current opinion is that they have no effect on the inflammatory aspect of asthma, despite being mast cell stabilizers. In fact a few studies have shown a deterioration in lung function with regular use (Spitzer et al, 1992; Wahedna et al, 1993). Many mechanisms have been put forward to explain a deleterious effect of continuous β_2-agonist usage (Warner, 1994). One possible explanation is that bronchodilatation allows inhalation of larger quantities of allergen and irritants, thereby increasing inflammation. Hence the present consensus that they be used only on an 'as required' basis. The recent introduction of long-acting β_2-agonists, with a duration of action of 12 hours, rather than the 4–6 hours of hitherto used preparations, has provided the scope for reducing the frequency of administration with better control of symptoms, especially at night. Their role in childhood asthma has yet to be fully established, but with more experience and long-term usage, they are likely to take over from the short-acting preparations as an adjuvant to anti-inflammatory drugs. The present recommendation for their use on a regular basis rather than as rescue medication also needs to be validated by long-term studies (Sears and Taylor, 1992) because of concern about the potential for a similar adverse effect as their short-acting equivalents.

Methylxanthines

This group of drugs is still widely used in North America but has fallen out of favour in most other countries, due to a narrow band of therapeutic effectiveness and potential for toxicity, leading to the need to monitor serum levels. The mechanism of action of this group of drugs is still not well understood, but the main effect seems to be to inhibit phosphodiesterase and thereby increase intracellular cyclic AMP. In addition to their bronchodilator effect, there is some evidence to show that they have an anti-inflammatory role in atopic asthma (Sullivan et al, 1994). Slow-release preparations are available with a duration of action beyond 12 hours, but carry with them the risk of significant fluctuations in plasma concentrations. Theophylline does have a role in an acute severe asthmatic attack where it may be given as a slow infusion.

Type IV phosphodiesterase inhibitors are being tested as more specific anti-asthma agents than the present methylxanthines and would work by increasing cyclic AMP levels in inflammatory cells and bronchial smooth muscle.

Antihistamines

These drugs do not have a major role to play as anti-asthmatic agents. However, newer selective H_1-antagonists which do not have the CNS effects, may have a limited role. Ketotifen is used by some clinicians in the management of the under 3 age group, where some benefits have been observed (Neijens and Knol, 1988; Likura et al, 1992). Furthermore, cetirizine has a down-regulatory effect on eosinophil migration probably via an effect on the ICAM-1 molecule (Fadel et al, 1987; Canonica et al, 1991). This may explain its weak anti-asthma effect which may be of greatest value as prophylaxis in infant wheezers.

New developments

Leukotriene antagonists are being actively developed as potent anti-inflammatory and bronchodilator agents, with encouraging preliminary results (Hui and Barnes, 1991; Taylor et al, 1991).

Phase 2 trials are being conducted into the role of PAF antagonists, having been shown to be potent inhibitors of PAF and allergen-induced bronchoconstriction and bronchial hyperresponsiveness in guinea-pigs (Roberts et al, 1988; Takizawa et al, 1988; Wilkens et al, 1990).

Newer immunosuppressants like cyclosporin A and FK506 are being tried in animal models and seem to have potent suppressant effects on T-cells, pro-inflammatory and inflammatory cells. A short-term clinical trial of cyclosporin has demonstrated its potential as a therapeutic agent in steroid-resistant very severe asthma (Alexander et al, 1992).

EVIDENCE OF AIRWAY INFLAMMATION IN CHILDHOOD ASTHMA

Most of the evidence for airway inflammation being a characteristic feature in asthma (Figure 3) comes from studies conducted in adults (Kay, 1991), using post-mortem examinations, bronchial biopsies (Dunnill, 1960; James et al, 1989; Laitenen et al, 1993), bronchoalveolar lavage (BAL) (De Monchy et al, 1985; Diaz et al, 1986; Wardlaw et al, 1988) and recently, sputum induction (Pin et al, 1992; Iredale et al, 1994). Similar studies in children present major problems, both for ethical and practical reasons, though a recent study by Ferguson et al (1992) did indeed reveal a corre-

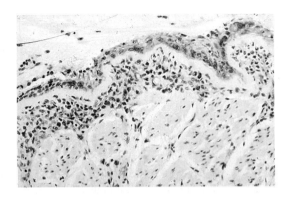

Figure 3. Histopathology of a bronchial biopsy in an adolescent with asthma, showing eosinophil infiltration and sub-basement membrane collagen deposition.

lation between bronchial eosinophil and mast cell activation and bronchial hyperresponsiveness in children. The use of bronchoscopies for research, the single procedure that has revolutionized our understanding of adult disease, is still considered unacceptable in children. Some evidence exists from ultrastructural examination of the airways of two asthmatic children undergoing open lung biopsies during clinical remission, compared with lung tissue of two children dying in status asthmaticus, all of whom had submucosal cellular infiltrates, especially with eosinophils, and denudation of epithelium (Cutz et al, 1978). It is salutary to note that these observations were made by paediatricians in 1978, some years before the seminal publication by Laitinen in 1985. Evidence has been collected of the correlation between BAL and serum levels of markers of eosinophil activation in adults (Adelroth et al, 1990), and their correlation with lung function (Bousquet et al, 1991; Broide et al, 1991) as well as a reduction in levels with anti-inflammatory treatment (Lee et al, 1984), thereby providing an additional measure of airway inflammation. Anecdotal evidence exists for the correlation of serum ECP and EPX with symptoms of asthma in the young child (Zimmerman et al, 1994). A significant difference has been demonstrated in serum ECP levels in asthmatic children with normal and decreased peak flow measurements (Hedlin et al, 1992). Boner et al (1993) have shown that changes in these serum markers correlate well with changes in airway function on allergen avoidance at high altitude. Our own studies show a good correlation between airway function and serum markers of eosinophil activation, both at baseline (Rao et al, 1994) (Figure. 4) and longitudinally over a period of 8 months, on institution of inhaled steroids (Figure 5), in a group of children with moderately severe asthma (Rao et al, unpublished data). As it is now well documented that steroids act by damping down the eosinophil mediated airway inflammation, these results provide good, if indirect, evidence of the pathology in the airways being similar to that in adult asthmatics.

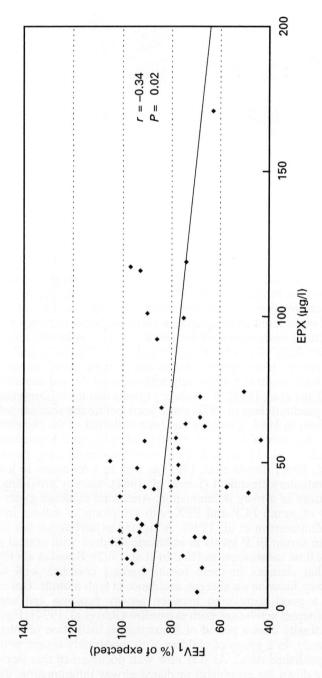

Figure 4. Correlation of serum EPX values with FEV₁ (percent of expected) in childhood asthma. (Forty-six children with moderate asthma.)

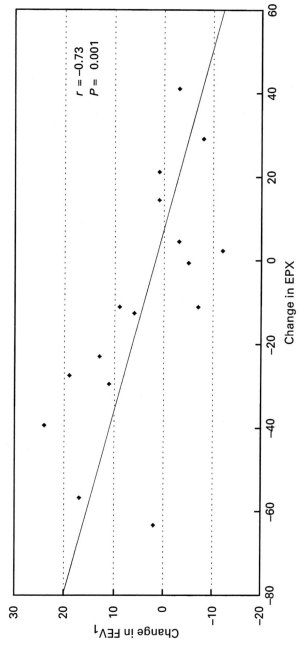

Figure 5. Correlation of percent change in serum EPX with percent change in FEV₁ in childhood asthma. (Sixteen asthmatic children followed over 8 months.)

ROLE OF INTERCURRENT VIRAL INFECTIONS IN ASTHMA

It has long been known that viral respiratory infections produce exacer-bations of wheeze in children. This is especially true of the under 5 years age group, and the tendency diminishes with age, with a high percentage apparently outgrowing their susceptibility. It has been thought that a severe viral infection in infancy, such as bronchiolitis, can trigger the process of asthma, but evidence is accumulating that infants who have a severe bronchiolitis are predisposed by virtue of having smaller calibre airways due to maternal smoking, lower birth weight, and the male sex. However, children with asthma (at any age) are predisposed to a large number of virus infections, which in turn produce an exacerbation. It is likely that the under-lying mechanisms of this interrelation are via the aggravation of airway inflammation (Busse, 1993). Studies carried out in different age groups of asthmatic children with clinical, microbiological and/or serological evidence of viral respiratory infections have revealed that approximately 40% of asthma exacerbations are associated with documented infections (McIntosh et al, 1973; Minor et al, 1974), rising to 70% when modern virus detection procedures are used (Johnston et al, 1993b). Bacterial infections did not have the same effect. These and subsequent studies have shown that a number of respiratory viruses can produce episodes of wheeze, and the relative incidence varies with age, with respiratory syncytial virus (RSV) being the commonest precipitant in the younger child and rhinovirus and influenza virus being more common in the older group (Horn and Gregg, 1973; Minor et al, 1976: Henderson et al, 1979). It appears that children with asthma have a higher rate of viral respiratory infections as well as more severe lower respiratory symptoms with them, compared to non-asthmatic controls (Isaacs et al, 1982).

Various mechanisms have been postulated to explain how viruses affect asthma. These include the production of virus-specific IgE antibodies, whose titres correlate to the extent of the infective processes (Welliver et al, 1991). The presence and level of specific IgE antibodies were found to be predictive of subsequent wheeze. In vitro studies have also shown that when leukocytes were incubated with respiratory viruses, an augmentation of basophil histamine release occurred (Ida et al, 1979; Busse et al, 1983), which was T-cell dependent (Huftel et al, 1992). This effect is probably mediated by the release of various cytokines, leading to enhancement of the inflammatory process. Studies by Busse et al (1993) have demonstrated that respiratory infections with rhinovirus enhance airway responsiveness, promote the development of a late asthmatic response and increase the air-way inflammatory response to antigen, probably mediated by release of cytokines. A recent paper by Balfour-Lynn et al (1994) showed a signifi-cant increase in tumour necrosis factor-α (TNF-α), a cytokine marker of local inflammation, in the nasal mucosa of children with virus-induced wheeze. Adenoviral infection can be associated with quite serious morbidity and chronic sequelae by virtue of its takeover of the host cell for replication of the viral genome and persistence long after the acute episode is over, and it is possible that continued stimulation of the immune system by the viral proteins maintains chronic allergic airway inflammation (Hogg, 1994; Macek et al, 1994).

INFANT WHEEZING VERSUS ASTHMA

A common problem facing paediatricians is the early diagnosis of asthma in the wheezing infant, the incidence of which is progressively rising. At least a third of children in the UK are known to wheeze in the first 5 years of life (Strachan, 1985). There seem to be two sub-groups of children, those who wheeze with viral respiratory infections and are asymptomatic in between episodes, and those who have a multitude of trigger factors, including viral infections, for wheezing, or have a chronic wheeze or cough. The latter group have an increased association with atopy. The episodic wheezers do not seem to have any such association and a majority 'grow out' of their wheezing problem (Park et al, 1986). A number of terms have been used for this group, such as 'wheezy bronchitis', 'happy wheezer' and 'post-bronchiolitic wheeze'. None of these accurately reflects the pathophysiology behind the wheezing, which may have quite a diverse aetiology. The vast majority of viral infections in this preschool age group are due to human rhinovirus, with an increased incidence of RSV in the first year of life, although many other respiratory viruses have been implicated (Carlson et al, 1984; Wright et al, 1989, Johnston et al, 1993a,b). A large number of children have only a few episodes of infection-induced wheeze but some have frequent episodes throughout the first two or three winters of life (Wilson, 1994). The incidence of atopic asthma, with chronic nocturnal cough and wheeze, increases with age (Zimmerman et al, 1988) usually after the age of 2–3 years, although the initial presentation may be with viral-induced episodic wheeze during infancy, thus making the distinction between the two extremely difficult. As yet there is a paucity of information on the pathophysiology at a cellular level for the different patterns of early wheezing. It is known, however, that infants who wheeze have a diminished lung function even prior to their first respiratory infection (Martinez et al, 1988, 1991). Prenatal influences on lung development, including maternal smoking, and genetic factors may play a role in wheezing starting in the first year (Camilli et al, 1993; Tager et al, 1993). These do not seem to be important factors for wheeze developing after the second year. The male gender also has a bearing on the early onset of wheeze (Martinez et al, 1991; Tager et al, 1993). No relationship has been detected between early wheeze and atopy (Sporik et al, 1991; Burr et al, 1993). With increasing age, the relationship develops and the severity of wheezing reflects the degree of allergic sensitization (Zimmerman et al, 1988). It is not known at what age the typical findings of chronic eosinophilic airway inflammation, found in adults, develop in the young child. Studies are needed to ascertain the differences between episodic viral wheeze and atopic wheeze at an early stage so that therapeutic intervention can be targeted before irreversible inflammatory changes of adult asthma become established.

EARLY ENVIRONMENTAL INFLUENCES

Fetal undernutrition during critical periods of development may have a lifelong effect on structure, function and metabolism of the individual (Rinas et al, 1993). This process of programming, occurring at different stages of gestation, has been linked to specific patterns of impaired and disproportionate fetal growth (Barker et al, 1993). Disproportionate babies may have average birth weights but a large head circumference and tend to have slow growth in infancy. These characteristics are associated with a tendency to develop atopy and an increased risk of death from obstructive airways disease as adults. Prospective studies also show that lower levels of neonatal lung function precede and predict episodes of wheezing in the first year (Martinez et al, 1991). A recent study showed a relationship between increasing head circumference at birth and higher levels of IgE in adult life, independent of gestational age and other confounding variables (Godfrey et al, 1994). A hypothesis to explain this finding is that fetal undernutrition late in gestation has a greater effect on the faster growing fetuses, evidenced by larger head size, with a redistribution of blood and nutrients to the brain at the expense of the trunk and limbs, resulting in a disproportionate fetus. This will lead to compromized thymic function and a decrease in Th_1 type lymphocytes and high levels of Th_2 cells, which sets the scene for the development of high IgE and atopic disease.

A number of studies have shown a relationship between parental, especially maternal, smoking and the development of atopic disease in the young child (Magnusson, 1986; Arshad et al, 1992), which may persist into later life (Ware et al, 1984). Other studies reveal that maternal smoking during pregnancy results in poorer lung function in the infant which predisposes to an increased incidence of early respiratory disease (Taylor and Wadsworth, 1987; Hanrahan et al, 1992), but not necessarily atopic asthma. However, maternal smoking in pregnancy is also associated with higher levels of IgE in the cord blood than is found in the offspring of nonsmoking mothers (Magnusson, 1986).

It is doubtful whether early infections, especially viral, increase the incidence of atopic asthma. It seems more likely that infants with a strong family history of atopy will develop IgE antibodies in response to the infection and go on to have atopic asthma (Welliver et al, 1980). There may, in fact, be an inverse relationship between infection and atopy, in that fewer early respiratory infections in children with no elder siblings increases their risk of developing atopy, compared with second and subsequent children in families (Strachan, 1989).

Our own studies suggest that the Th_2 phenotype is already present at birth. It is possible to identify that infants, who develop recurrent wheezing and a positive skin test to cat fur by 1 year of age, already have at birth cord blood mononuclear cells which fail to release IFN-γ under stimulation with cat fur extract. This indicates that sensitization and subversion to a Th_2 phenotype have occurred antenatally, presumably via the mother. Maternal factors such as poor nutrition, smoking and atopy probably influence this.

Postnatally, high aeroallergen exposure will draw the sensitized lymphocytes into the airway mucosa, thus setting up airway inflammation. This raises the possibility that early allergen avoidance may prevent the development of the disease.

SUMMARY

It is clear that in established childhood asthma the airway immuno-pathology is similar, if not identical, to that which exists in adult asthma. However, as this evolves through early childhood, there are stages when the process is reversible. Once a vicious cycle of self-perpetuating inflammation has developed, only relatively blunderbuss treatment, such as high dose inhaled and oral steroids, will have any significant impact. Furthermore, when extensive epithelial shedding has led to repair by sub basement-membrane fibrosis, it is likely that a degree of airflow limitation will be irreversible.

Intervention at an early stage when lymphocytes first appear in the airways, or when eosinophilic inflammation is just beginning to evolve, may be effective even using drugs with little efficacy in established disease, such as antihistamines. Better responses in young children with allergic asthma to sodium cromoglycate and other nonsteroidal disease modifying agents may also be explained by this mechanism.

Once further insights have been gained into the ontogeny of airway inflammation, without a doubt therapeutic strategies will be significantly altered. However, caution is required in extrapolating the results of therapeutic trials in older children to infancy where the majority of wheezers do not develop chronic atopic asthma.

REFERENCES

Adelroth E, Rosenhall L, Johansson S-A, et al (1990) Inflammatory cells and eosinophil activity in asthmatics investigated by bronchoalveolar lavage: the effects of anti asthma treatment with budesonide or terbutaline. *American Review of Respiratory Diseases* **142:** 91–99.

Alexander AG, Barnes NC & Kay AB (1992) Trial of cyclosporin in corticosteroid-dependent chronic severe asthma. *Lancet* **339:** 324–328.

Alving K, Matran R, Lacroix JS et al (1990) Capsaicin and histamineantagonist sensitive mechanisms in the immediate allergic reaction of pig airways. *Acta Physiologica Scandinavica* **138:** 49–60.

Amelung PJ, Panhuysen CIM, Postma DS et al (1992) Atopy, asthma and bronchial hyper-responsiveness: exclusion of linkage to markers on chromosome *11q and 6p. Clinical and Experimental Allergy* **22:** 1077–1084.

Arshad SH, Matthews S, Grant C & Hide DW (1992) Effects of allergen avoidance on development of allergic disorders in infancy. *Lancet* **339:** 1493–1497.

Balfour-Lynn IM, Valman HB, Wellings R et al (1994) Tumour necrosis factor-alpha and leukotriene E$_4$ production in wheezy infants. *Clinical and Experimental Allergy* **24:** 121–126.

Bard PR, Rogers HW, Gordon JR et al (1989) IL-3 dependent and independent mast cells stimulated with IgE express multiple cytokines. *Journal of Experimental Medicine* **170:** 245.

Barker DJP, Gluckman PD, Godfrey KM et al (1993) Fetal nutrition and cardiovascular disease in adult life. *Lancet* **341:** 938–941.

Beasley R, Roche WR, Roberts JA & Holgate ST (1989) Cellular events in the bronchi in mild asthma and after bronchial provocation. *American Review of Respiratory Diseases* **139:** 806–817.

Bentley AM, Menz G, Storz C et al (1992) Identification of T-lymphocytes, macrophages and activated eosinophils in the bronchial mucosa in intrinsic asthma: Relationship to symptoms and broncial hyperresponsiveness. *American Review of Respiratory Diseases* **146:** 500–506.

Blumenthal MN, Namboodiri K, Mendell N et al (1981) Genetic transmission of serum IgE levels. *American Journal of Medical Genetics* **10:** 219–228.

Boner AL, Peroni DG, Piacentini GL & Venge P (1993) Influence of allergy avoidance at high altitude on serum markers of eosinophil activation in children with asthma. *Clinical and Experimental Allergy* **23:** 1021–1026.

Borecki IB, Rao DC, Lalouel JM et al (1985) Demonstration of a common major gene with pleiotropic effects on immunoglobulin E levels and allergy. *Genetic Epidemiology* **2:** 327–338.

Bousquet J, Chanez P, Lacoste JY et al (1990) Eosinophilic inflammation in asthma. *New England Journal of Medicine* **323:** 1033–1039.

Bousquet J, Chanez P, Lacoste JY et al (1991) Indirect evidence of bronchial inflammation assessed by titration of inflammatory mediators in BAL fluid of patients with asthma. *Journal of Allergy and Clinical Immunology* **88:** 649–660.

Broide DH, Gleich GJ, Cuomo AJ et al (1991) Evidence of ongoing mast cell and eosinophil degranulation in symptomatic asthma airway. *Journal of Allergy and Clinical Immunology* **88:** 637–648.

Burr ML, Butland BK, King S & Vaughan-Williams E (1989) Changes in asthma prevalence: two surveys 15 years apart. *Archives of Diseases of Childhood* **64:** 1452–1456.

Burr ML, Limb ES, Maguire MJ et al (1993) Infant feeding, wheezing and allergy: a prospective study. *Archives of Diseases of Childhood* **68:** 724–728.

Busse WW (1993) Role and contribution of viral respiratory infections to asthma. *Allergy* **48:** 57–61.

Busse WW, Swenson CA, Borden EC et al (1983) The effect of influenza A virus on leukocyte histamine release. *Journal of Allergy and Clinical Immunology* **71:** 382–388.

Busse WW, Lemanske Jr RF, Stark JM & Calhoun WJ (1993) The role of respiratory infections in Asthma. In Holgate ST, Austen KF, Lichtenstein LM & Kay AB (eds) *Asthma: Physiology, Immunopharmacology and Treatment. Fourth International Symposium*, pp 345–355. London: Academic Press.

Camilli AE, Holberg CJ, Wright AL & Taussig LM (1993) Parental childhood respiratory illness and respiratory illness in their infants. *Pediatric Pulmonology* **16:** 275–280.

Canonica GW, Parodi MN, Boero F et al (1991) Effects of cetirizine and deflazacort on cell adhesion molecules expression on lymphocytes and epithelial cells. *Schweizerische Medizinische Wochenschrift* **121:** 38.

Carlson KH, Orstavik I, Leergard J & Hoeg H (1984) Respiratory virus infections and aeroallergens in acute bronchial asthma. *Archives of Diseases of Childhood* **59:** 310–315.

Cookson WOC, Sharp PA, Faux JA & Hopkin JM (1989) Linkage between immunoglobulin E responses, underlying asthma and rhinitis, and chromosome *11q. Lancet* **i:** 1292–1295.

Cutz F, Levison H & Cooper DM (1978) Ultrastructure of airways in children with asthma. *Histopathology* **2:** 407–421.

De Monchy JG, Kauffman HF, Venge P et al (1985) Bronchoalveolar eosinophils during allergen-induced late asthmatic reactions. *American Review of Respiratory Diseases* **131:** 373–376.

Diaz P, Gonzalez C, Galleguillos F, et al (1986) Eosinophils and macrophages in bronchial mucus and bronchoalveolar lavage during allergen induced late-phase reactions. *Journal of Allergy and Clinical Immunology* **77:** S244.

Diaz P, Gonzalez MC, Galleguillos FR et al (1989) Leukocytes and mediators in BAL during allergen-induced late-phase asthmatic reactions. *American Review of Respiratory Diseases* **139:** 1383–1389.

Dunnill MS (1960) The pathology of asthma with special reference to changes in the bronchial mucosa. *Journal of Clinical Pathology* **13:** 27–33.

Dunnill MS (1978) The pathology of asthma. In Middleton E, Reed CE & Ellis EE (eds) *Allergy, Principles and Practice*, pp 678–686. St Louis: CV Mosby.

Dunnill MS, Massarella GR & Anderson JA (1969) A comparison of the quantitive anatomy of the bronchi in normal subjects and status asthmaticus in chronic bronchitis and in emphysema. *Thorax* **24:** 176–179.

Fadel R, Herpin-Richard N, Rihoux JP & Henocq E (1987) Inhibitory effect of cetirizine 2HCl on eosinophil migration in vivo. *Clinics in Allergy* **17:** 373–379.

Ferguson AC, Whitelaw M & Brown H (1992) Correlation of bronchial eosinophil and mast cell activation with bronchial hyperresponsiveness in children with asthma. *Journal of Allergy and Clinical Immunology* **90:** 606–613.

Florey HW (1962) Secretion of mucus in the inflammation of mucus membranes. In Florey H (ed.) *General Pathology*, pp 167–196. London: Lloyd Luke Medical Books Ltd.

Frick WE, Sedgewick JB & Busse WW (1989) The appearance of hypodense eosinophils in antigen dependent late phase asthma. *American Review of Respiratory Diseases* **139:** 1401–1406.

Gauchet JF, Lebman DA, Coffman RL et al (1990) Structure and expression of germline E transcripts in human B-cells induced by interleukin-4 to switch to IgE production. *Journal of Experimental Medicine* **172:** 463–473.

Gemou-Engesaeth V, Kay AB, Bush A & Corrigan CJ (1994) Activated peripheral blood CD4 and CD8 T-lymphocytes in child asthma: correlation with eosinophilia and disease severity. *Paediatric Allergy and Immunology* **5:** 170–177.

Gleich GJ, Frigas E, Langering DA et al (1979) Cytotoxic properties of eosinophil major basic protein. *Journal of Immunology* **123:** 2925.

Godfrey KM, Barker DJP & Osmond C (1994) Disproportionate foetal growth and raised immunoglobulin E concentration in adult life. *Clinical and Experimental Allergy* **24:** 641–648.

Hallgren R & Venge P (1991) The eosinophil in inflammation. In Matsson P & Venge P (eds) *Clinical Impact of the Monitoring of Allergic Inflammation in Asthma*, pp 119–140. London: Academic Press.

Hanrahan JP, Tager IRA, Segal B et al (1992) The effect of maternal smoking during pregnancy on early infant lung function. *American Review of Respiratory Diseases* **145:** 1129–1135.

Hanson B, McGue M, Roitman-Johnson B et al (1991) Atopic disease and immunoglobulin E in twins reared apart and together. *American Journal of Human Genetics* **48:** 873–879.

Hasstedt SJ, Meyers DA & Marsh DG (1983) Inheritance of immunoglobulin E: genetic model fitting. *American Journal of Medical Genetics* **14:** 61–66.

Hedlin G, Ahlstedt S, Hakansson L & Venge P (1992) Levels in serum of ECP, eosinophil chemotactic activity (ECA), and tryptase before and during bronchial challenge in cat allergic children with asthma. *Pediatric Allergy and Immunology* **3:** 144–149.

Henderson FW, Clyde WA, Collier AM et al (1979) The etiology and epidemiologic spectrum of bronchiolitis in pediatric practice. *Journal of Pediatrics* **95:** 183.

Hogg JC (1994) Adenoviral infection and childhood asthma. *American Journal of Respiratory and Critical Care Medicine* **150:** 2–3.

Horn MEC & Gregg I (1973) Role of viral infection and host factors in acute episodes of asthma and chronic bronchitis. *Chest* **63:** 44–47.

Holgate ST & Church MK (1993) Asthma—Pathophysiology. In Holgate ST & Church MK (eds) *Allergy*, pp 13.1–13.12. London: Gower Medical Publishing.

Holgate ST, Robinson C & Church MK (1988) Mediators of immediate hypersensitivity. In Middleton E, Reid CE, Ellis EF et al (eds) *Allergy, Principles and Practice*, pp 135–136. Washington DC: Mosby.

Holt PG (1993). Regulation of antigen presenting cell functions in lung and airway tissue. *European Respiratory Journal* **6:** 120–129.

Hossain S & Heard BE (1970) Hyperplasia of bronchial muscle in asthma. *Journal of Pathology* **101:** 171–184.

Huftel MA, Swenson CA, Borcherding WR et al (1992) The effect of T-cell depletion on enhanced basophil histamine release after in vitro incubation with live influenza virus. *American Journal of Respiration and Cellular Molecular Biology* **7:** 434–440.

Hui KP & Barnes NC (1991) Lung function improvement in asthma with a cysteinyl-leukotriene antagonist. *Lancet* **337:** 1062–1063.

Ida S, Hooks JJ, Siraganian RP & Notkens AL (1979) Enhancement of IgE mediated histamine release from human basophil by viruses: Role of interferon. *Journal of Experimental Medicine* **145:** 892–896.

Iredale MJ, Wanklyn SAR, Phillips IP, et al (1994) Non-invasive assessment of bronchial inflammation in asthma: no correlation between eosinophilia of induced sputum and broncial hyperresponsiveness to inhaled hypertonic saline. *Clinical and Experimental Allergy* **24:** 940–946.

Isaacs D, Clarke JR, Tyrrell DAJ & Valman HB (1982) Selective infection of lower respiratory tract by respiratory viruses in children with recurrent respiratory tract infections. *British Medical Journal* **284:** 1746–1748.

James AL, Pare PD & Hogg JC (1989) The mechanics of airway narrowing in asthma. *American Review of Respiratory Diseases* **139**: 242–246.

Johnston SL, Bardin PG & Pattemore PK (1993a) Viruses as precipitants of asthma III. Rhinoviruses: molecular biology and prospects for future intervention. *Clinical and Experimental Allergy* **23**: 237–246.

Johnston SL, Sanderson G, Pattemore PK et al (1993b) Use of polymerase chain reaction for diagnosis of picornavirus infection in subjects with and without respiratory symptoms. *Journal of Clinical Microbiology* **31**: 111–117.

Kay AB (1991) Asthma and inflammation. *Journal of Allergy and Clinical Immunology* **87**: 893–900.

Laitinen LA, Heino M, Laitinen A et al (1985) Damage to the airway epithelium and bronchial reactivity in patients with asthma. *American Review of Respiratory Diseases* **131**: 599–606.

Laitinen LA, Laitinen A & Haahtela T (1993) Airway mucosal inflammation even in patients with newly diagnosed asthma. *American Review of Respiratory Diseases* **147**: 697–704.

Lee TC, Lenihan OJ, Malone B et al (1984) Increased synthesis of PAF in activated human eosinophils. *Journal of Biological Chemistry* **259**: 5526–5530.

Likura Y, Naspitz CK, Mikawa H et al (1992) Prevention of asthma by ketotifen in infants with atopic dermatitis. *Annals of Allergy* **68**: 233–236.

Lopez AF, Sanderson CJ, Gamble JR et al (1988) Recombinant IL-5 is a selective activator of human eosinophil function. *Journal of Experimental Medicine* **167**: 219–224.

Lubs EML (1972) Empiric risks for genetic counselling in families with allergy. *Journal of Pediatrics* **80**: 26–31.

Lympany P, Welsh K, McCochrane GM et al (1992) Genetic analysis using DNA polymorphism of the linkage between chromosome *11q13* and atopy and bronchial hyperresponsiveness to methacholine. *Journal of Allergy and Clinical Immunology* **88**: 619–628.

Macek V, Sorli J, Kopriva S & Marin J (1994) Persistent adenoviral infection and chronic airway obstruction in children. *American Journal of Respiratory and Critical Care Medicine* **150**: 7–10.

McIntosh K, Ellis EF, Hoffman LS et al (1973) The association of viral and bacterial infections with exacerbations of wheezing in young asthmatic children. *Journal of Pediatrics* **83**: 578–590.

Magnusson CG (1986) Maternal smoking affects cord serum IgE levels and increases the risk of subsequent infant allergy. *Journal of Allergy and Clinical Immunology* **78**: 898–904.

Marsh DG, Neely JD, Breazeale DR et al (1994) Linkage analysis of IL-4 and other chromosome *5q31.1* markers and total serum IgE concentrations. *Science* **264**: 1152–1156.

Martinez FD, Morgan WJ, Wright AL et al (1988) Diminished lung function as a predisposing factor for wheezing respiratory illness in infants. *New England Journal of Medicine* **319**: 1112–1117.

Martinez FD, Morgan WJ, Wright AL et al (1991) Initial airway function is a risk factor for recurrent wheezing respiratory illness during the first three years of life. *American Review of Respiratory Diseases* **143**: 312–316.

Minor TE, Dick EC, DeMeo AN et al (1974) Viruses as precipitants of asthmatic attacks in children. *Journal of the American Medical Association* **227**: 292–298.

Minor TE, Dick EC, Baker JW et al (1976) Rhinovirus and influenza A infections as precipitants of asthma. *American Review of Respiratory Diseases* **113**: 149–153.

Naylor B (1962) The shedding of the mucosa of the bronchial tree in asthma. *Thorax* **17**: 69–72.

Neijens HJ & Knol K (1988) Oral prophylactic treatment in wheezy infants. *Journal of Immunology and Allergy Practice* **10**: 17–23.

Nilsson G, Alving K, Anstedt S et al (1990) Peptidergic innervation of rat lymphoid tissue and lung—Relation to mast cell and sensitivity to capsaicin. *Cell and Tissue Research* **262**: 125–133.

Ninan TK & Russell G (1992) Respiratory symptoms and atopy in Aberdeen school children: evidence from two surveys 25 years apart. *British Medical Journal* **304**: 873–875.

Osler W (1892) Bronchial asthma. In *Principles and Practices of Medicine*, (1st edn., pp 497–501. New York: Appleton and Co.

Owen WF, Rothenberg ME, Silberstein DS et al (1987) Regulation of human eosinophil viability, density, and function by GM-CSF in the presence of 3T3 fibroblasts. *Journal of Experimental Medicine* **166**: 129–141.

Park ES, Golding J, Carswell F & Stewart-Brown S (1986) Pre-school wheezing and prognosis at 10. *Archives of Diseases of Childhood* **61**: 642–646.

Pin I, Gibson PG, Kolendowicz R et al (1992) Use of induced sputum cell counts to investigate airway inflammation in asthma. *Thorax* **47**: 28–29.

Raeburn JA (1990) Asthma and other allergic conditions. In Emery AE & Remoin DL (eds) *Principles and Practice of Medical Genetics*, pp 1173–1178. Edinburgh: Churchill Livingstone.

Rao KR, Hegarty J, Gregson RK et al (1994) Correlation between eosinophil markers of airway inflammation and parameters of airway function in childhood asthma. *European Respiratory Journal* **7:** 27s.

Rich SS, Roitman-Johnson B, Greenberg B et al (1992) Genetic analysis of atopy in three large kindreds: no evidence of linkage to *D11S97*. *Clinical and Experimental Allergy* **22:** 1070–1076.

Rinas U, Horneff G & Wahn V (1993) Interferon gamma production by cord blood mononuclear cells is reduced in newborns with a family history of atopic disease and is independent from cord blood IgE levels. *Paediatric Allergy and Immunology* **4:** 60–64.

Roberts NM, Page CP, Chung KF & Barnes PJ (1988) Effect of a PAF antagonist, BN 52063, on antigen-induced acute and late-onset cutaneous responses in atopic subjects. *American Review of Respiratory Diseases* **137:** 1317.

Roche WR, Beasley R, Williams JH & Holgate ST (1989) Subepithelial fibrosis in the bronchi of asthmatics. *Lancet* **ii:** 520–524.

Romagnani S (1992) Induction of Th$_1$ and Th$_2$ responses: a key role for the 'natural' immune response? *Immunology Today* **13:** 379–381.

Scott P (1993) IL-12: Initiation cytokine for cell mediated immunity. *Science* **260:** 496–497.

Sears MR & Taylor DR (1992) Regular beta-agonist therapy—the quality of the evidence. *European Respiratory Journal* **5:** 896–897.

Sears MR, Burrows B, Flannery EM et al (1993) Atopy in childhood. I. Gender and allergen related risks for development of hayfever and asthma. *Clinical and Experimental Allergy* **23:** 941–948.

Shaw RA, Crane J, O'Connell TV et al (1990) Increasing prevalence of asthma in a rural New Zealand adolescent population 1975–1989. *Archives of Diseases of Childhood* **65:** 1319–1323.

Shaw RJ, Cromwell O & Kay AB (1984) Preferential generation of leukotriene C$_4$ by human eosinophils. *Clinical and Experimental Immunology* **56:** 716–722.

Sheffer AL (chairman, international asthma project) (1992). *International consensus report on the diagnosis and management of asthma.* Publication 92–3091. National Heart, Lung and Blood Institute, National Institutes of Health, Bethseda, Maryland.

Sobonya RE (1984) Concise clinical study: Quantitive changes in long-standing allergic asthma. *American Review of Respiratory Diseases* **130:** 289–292.

Spitzer WO, Suissa S, Ernst P et al (1992) The use of beta-agonists and the risk of death and near-death from asthma. *New England Journal of Medicine* **326:** 501–506.

Sporik R, Holgate ST & Cogswell JJ (1991) Natural history of asthma in childhood—a birth cohort study. *Archives of Diseases of Childhood* **66:** 1050–1053.

Strachan DP (1985) The prevalence and natural history of wheezing in early childhood. *Journal of the Royal College of General Practitioners* **35:** 182–184.

Strachan DP (1989) Hay fever, hygiene and household size. *British Medical Journal* **299:** 1259–1260.

Sullivan P, Bekir S, Jaffar Z et al (1994) Anti-inflammatory effects of low dose oral theophylline in atopic asthma. *Lancet* **343:** 1006–1008.

Tager IB, Hanrahan JP, Tosteson TD et al (1993) Lung function, pre- and post-natal smoke exposure, and wheezing in the first year of life. *American Review of Respiratory Diseases* **147:** 811–817.

Takagi M, Nakahata T, Kenichi K et al (1989) Stimulation of connective tissue-type mast cell proliferation by cross linking of cell bound IgE. *Journal of Experimental Medicine* **170:** 233.

Takizawa H, Ishii A, Suzuki S et al (1988) Bronchoconstriction induced by platelet-activating factor in the guinea pig and its inhibition by CV-3988, a PAF antagonist: serial changes in findings of lung histology and bronchoalveolar lavage cell population. *International Archives of Allergy Applied Immunology* **86:** 375.

Taylor B & Wadsworth J (1987) Maternal smoking during pregnancy and lower respiratory tract illness in early life. *Archives of Diseases of Childhood* **62:** 786–791.

Taylor IK, O'Shaughnessy KM, Fuller R & Dollery CT (1991) Effect of cysteinyl-leukotriene receptor antagonist ICI 204.219 on allergen-induced bronchoconstriction and airway hyperreactivity in atopic subjects. *Lancet* **337:** 690–694.

Venge P & Peterson CGB (1989) Eosinophil biochemistry and killing mechanisms. In Morley J & Colditz I (eds) *Eosinophils in Asthma*, pp 163–177. London: Academic Press.

Wahedna I, Wong CS, Wisnieswki AFZ et al (1993) Asthma control during and after regular beta-agonist treatment. *American Review of Respiratory Diseases* **148:** 707.

Wardlaw AJ, Dunnette S, Gleich GJ et al (1988) Eosinophils and mast cells in bronchoalveolar lavage in subjects with mild asthma. *American Review of Respiratory Diseases* **137:** 62–69.

Ware JH, Dockery DW, Spiro FE & Ferris BG (1984) Passive smoking, gas cooking and respiratory health of children living in six cities. *American Review of Respiratory Diseases* **129**: 366–374

Warner JO (1993a) Impact on the quality of management of asthmatic children by monitoring of inflammation. *Allergy* **48**: 158–161.

Warner JO (1993b) Use of corticosteroids in children with asthma. *European Respiratory Review* **3**: 326–328.

Warner JO (1994) The beta$_2$-agonist controversy and its relevance to the treatment of children. *European Respiratory Review* **4**: 21–26.

Warner JO & Warner JA (1993) Paediatric allergy. In Lachmann PJ, Peters DK, Rosen FS & Walport MJ (eds) *Clinical Aspects of Immunology*, vol.2, pp 1081–1103. Oxford: Blackwell Scientific Publication.

Warner JO, Neifens HJ, Kinderzienhaus S et al (1992) Asthma: a follow-up statement from an International Paediatric Asthma Consensus Group. *Archives of Diseases of Childhood* **67**: 240–248.

Welliver RC, Kaul TN & Ogra PL (1980) The appearance of cell-bound IgE in respiratory epithelium after respiratory-syncytial-virus infection. *New England Journal of Medicine* **303**: 1198–1202.

Welliver RC, Wong DT, Sun M et al (1991) The development of respiratory syncytial virus specific IgE and the release of histamine in nasopharyngeal secretions after infection. *New England Journal of Medicine* **305**: 841–846.

Wiggs BR, Bosken C, Pare PD et al (1992) A model of airway narrowing in asthma and in chronic obstructive pulmonary disease. *American Review of Respiratory Diseases* **145**: 1251–1258.

Wilkens JH, Wilkens H, Uffman J et al (1990) Effect of a PAF antagonist (BN 52063) on broncho-constriction and platelet activation during exercise induced asthma. *British Journal of Clinical Pharmacology* **85**: 85–92.

Wilson NM (1994) The significance of early wheezing. *Clinical and Experimental Allergy* **24**: 522–529.

Wright AL, Taussig LM, Ray CG et al (1989) The Tucson childrens respiratory study. II Lower respiratory tract illness in the first year of life. *American Journal of Epidemiology* **129**: 1232–1246.

Yamaguchi Y, Hayashi Y, Sugama Y et al (1988) Highly purified murine IL-5 stimulates eosinophil function and prolongs in vitro survival. *Journal of Experimental Medicine* **167**: 1737–1742.

Zimmerman B, Fearney S, Reisman et al (1988) Allergy in asthma. I. The dose relationship of allergy to severity of childhood asthma. *Journal of Allergy and Clinical Immunology* **81**: 63–70.

Zimmerman B, Enander I, Zimmerman R & Ahlstedt S (1994) Asthma in children under 5 years of age: eosinophils and serum levels of eosinophil proteins ECP and EPX in relation to atopy and symptoms. *Clinical and Experimental Allergy* **24**: 149–155.

4

Wheezing in infants and its relation to asthma

FERNANDO D. MARTINEZ

The relation between wheezing lower respiratory illnesses (LRI) occurring in early childhood and the subsequent development of asthma has been the matter of considerable discussion during the last 40 years. In 1953, Boesen (Boesen, 1953) reported the results of the earliest follow-up study of children who had 'asthmatic bronchitis' in early life. He mailed questionnaires to the parents of children from Copenhagen hospitalized with this diagnosis 6–11 years earlier. He observed that only 3% of infants admitted during the first 6 months of life had 'regular attacks of asthma' at follow-up compared with 7% of those admitted between 6 and 11 months, 18% of those admitted between 12 and 35 months and 42% of those admitted after the age of 3. Boesen also reported that, among Copenhagen schoolchildren aged 7–14 years, prevalence of asthma was 0.8% in 1949–1950. This study thus suggested a connection between acute respiratory illnesses requiring hospitalization in early life and the subsequent development of asthma. It also showed that prognosis was better for episodes occurring in the first year of life.

Many subsequent studies have confirmed that children who wheeze during viral infections in early life are at increased risk of developing asthma (reviewed by Samet et al, 1983), but the factors responsible for this connection are not yet entirely understood. Two main approaches to this problem have been proposed (Morgan, 1990). Many investigators consider wheezing a manifestation of a condition, or conditions, that pre-exist the viral infection which usually provokes the illness. Others assume that viral infections may prime the immune system, damage the lungs, and cause a substantial alteration in airway function, all of which may predispose the infant to persistent bronchial responsiveness and to the subsequent development of asthma. Unfortunately, most studies of the outcome of wheezing in early life are based on small numbers of selected subjects or on subjects who were enrolled in the early school years and in whom the history of wheezing during infancy was obtained retrospectively. Only recently have the results of a few prospective studies initiated at birth (Wright et al, 1989) or during infancy (Strope et al, 1991) become available. These studies have considerably changed our understanding of this issue and will be the focus of this chapter.

Baillière's Clinical Paediatrics —
Vol. 3, No. 2, May 1995
ISBN 0–7020–1986–0

WHEEZING ILLNESSES IN INFANCY AND LUNG FUNCTION

Several prospective studies have shown that infants with a history of bronchiolitis or wheezing have persistently lower levels of several indices of lung function measured many years later. Sims et al (1978) studied 8-year-old children who had proven respiratory syncytial virus (RSV) bronchiolitis in infancy and found that they had diminished lung function when compared to controls. Pullen and Hey (1982) assessed lung function in 130 children 10 years after hospitalization for RSV-LRI occurring during infancy and found that these children had significantly lower mean values for several indices derived from the maximal expiratory flow-volume curve than controls. Mok and Simpson (1982) followed 200 8-year-old children who had been hospitalized for bronchiolitis during infancy. They found that these children had approximately 5% lower forced expiratory volume in the first second (FEV_1) and 12% lower mean forced expiratory flow between 25% and 75% of vital capacity (FEF_{25-75}) than children without a history of bronchiolitis.

It is apparent that all these initial studies were performed in children who were hospitalized for LRI in early life. In could be argued that these children may have a more severe expression of the same disease affecting other children who do not require hospitalization. It is also possible that most infants who require hospitalization may have a disease altogether, distinct from that affecting infants with milder illnesses. Strope et al (1991) studied the relation between mild LRI not requiring hospitalization, as documented by the children's paediatricians during the first 6 years of life, and lung function assessed at age 6–18 years in 89 boys and 70 girls. They found that boys who had experienced two or more episodes of wheezing LRI during the preschool years had lower FEV_1 and FEF_{25-75}, among other lung function parameters, than did boys with one or less wheezing illnesses or who had nonwheezing illnesses. The association between preschool wheezing LRIs and lower subsequent lung function was also present among girls, but did not reach statistical significance probably because of the smaller number of girls involved. The study by Strope et al (1991) thus demonstrated that diminished lung function levels subsequent to wheezing LRIs were not exclusive of subjects with more severe wheezing illnesses requiring hospitalization in early life.

The pathophysiological mechanisms responsible for these diminished levels of lung function have been the matter of considerable debate. It was understood from the beginning that it was unlikely that persistence of symptoms could be the only explanation for these findings, because diminished lung function was also observed among subjects who had been symptom-free after early childhood (Strope et al, 1991). It remained to be elucidated if the lower levels of lung function observed in infants with wheezing LRIs were inborn or were otherwise induced by the viral infections themselves.

Three studies contributed to clarify this issue, at least in part (Martinez et al, 1991; Tager et al, 1993; Young et al, 1994). Investigators in Tucson and Boston in the U.S., and in Perth in Australia took advantage of the development of new techniques to assess lung function in infancy (Taussig et al, 1982), and obtained data for maximal expiratory flows at end-tidal expiration ($\dot{V}_{max}$FRC) during the first 6 months of life and before any LRI developed. There has been considerable debate about what aspect of lung function $\dot{V}_{max}$FRC represents, but studies using bronchodilators and histamine have demonstrated a pattern of responses that suggest that $\dot{V}_{max}$FRC reflects the size of the intrathoracic airways (Prendiville et al, 1987). The studies by Martinez et al (1991), Tager et al (1993) and Young et al (1994) showed convincingly that infants who would subsequently develop wheezing illnesses had, as a group, lower mean $\dot{V}_{max}$FRC before any such illness developed.

These studies gave rise to the hypothesis that, in many if not most instances, infant wheezing could be a mechanical phenomenon, associated with a critically smaller airway diameter (Martinez et al, 1988). Briefly stated this hypothesis suggests that both genetic and intrauterine factors determine the size of the intrapulmonary bronchi at birth. This size is a function of the size of the lung, of the thickness of the airway wall, and of the forces that keep airways void of cartilage open (Martinez et al, 1991). Wheezing is the vibration induced by the passage of air through an airway after a critical resistance to airflow in the lumen of that airway has been reached. Because resistance is a function of the fourth power of the radius, reductions in airway diameter due to oedema, mucus, and intraluminal fluid may result in markedly higher increases in resistance in airways with diminished initial intraluminal diameters.

This hypothesis offered a plausible explanation for the changes in the incidence of wheezing illnesses with age: this incidence is highest in the first months of life and decreases markedly after 6 months of age (Martinez, in press). Morgan and Martinez (unpublished observations) recently showed that maximal flows grow faster than lung volumes during the first 6 years of life and it is thus likely that the critical resistance for the development of wheezing may not be reached as easily in older children as it is in infants.

WHEEZING IN INFANCY AND BRONCHIAL HYPERRESPONSIVENESS

In spite of these advances in our understanding of the risk factors for infant wheezing, several issues remained to be elucidated. The finding of diminished lung function prior to any LRI in children who subsequently developed wheezing LRIs did not clarify what causes these diminished airway function levels and, specifically, if bronchial hyperresponsiveness (BHR) and/or increased airway tone are involved in it. Indeed, it has been suggested that BHR may be a risk factor for wheezing LRIs in early life (Wilson et al, 1992). Several studies had found that children hospitalized with bronchiolitis in infancy had both higher prevalence of BHR and lower levels of lung function than children without such a history (Gurwitz et al, 1981; Sims et al, 1981; Pullen and Hey, 1982). More recently, three groups of researchers studied bronchial responsiveness to histamine or methacholine in infants with a history of bronchiolitis (Tepper et al, 1992) or who had wheezing episodes during the first months of life (Stick et al, 1991; Clarke et al, 1992). Tepper et al (1992) studied 18 infants with acute bronchiolitis, nine of whom were hospitalized for their disease, and 24 controls. They found that approximately 4 months after their illness, infants with bronchiolitis had significantly diminished percent predicted $\dot{V}_{max}FRC$ but bronchial responsiveness was not increased when compared to that of controls. Ten months after the acute episode, children with a history of bronchiolitis still had significantly diminished $\dot{V}_{max}FRC$ levels, but now their bronchial responsiveness was also significantly increased compared to controls. The authors proposed the hypothesis that most infants are born with BHR and become hyporesponsive with age, but in those who develop bronchiolitis, BHR may be more likely to persist. Both Stick et al (1991) and Clarke et al (1992) studied infants with a history of recurrent wheezing, and Stick et al specifically excluded infants with a diagnosis of RSV infection. Both groups reported lower $\dot{V}_{max}FRC$ levels in wheezy infants than in controls, but found no difference in level of bronchial responsiveness between the two groups. These results were in agreement with those reported by Voter et al (1988). These researchers studied lung function (using flow-volume curves) and methacholine responsiveness in 57 males between the ages of 11 and 22. These subjects belonged to the same paediatric practice in North Carolina on which Strope et al (1991) based their previously quoted study, and LRI history had been documented in the children's charts. Practically all LRIs were managed on an out-patient basis. The authors found no relation between preschool wheezing illness experience and methacholine sensitivity in these adolescent subjects, but they confirmed in this smaller subgroup of subjects that spirometric performance was significantly lower in children with two or more wheezing illnesses in early life.

It thus appears that, when studies are limited to subjects with mild diseases not requiring hospitalization, a consistent pattern of diminished levels of lung function but prevalence of BHR within normal ranges was observed, whether lung function tests or tests of bronchial responsiveness were performed months or years after the initial episode. Subjects with more severe symptoms requiring hospitalization also showed diminished average lung function parameters, but in several studies they showed increased prevalence of BHR as well. It remained to be elucidated if in these children, persistent BHR represented a hereditary developmental pattern attributable to an asthmatic predisposition or if it was the result of the viral insult itself. In a study of 63 normal infants without a history of LRI, Young et al (1991) assessed bronchial responsiveness to histamine at a mean age of 4.5 weeks, and thus before LRIs had occurred. They found that subjects with a family history of asthma had similar baseline $\dot{V}_{max}FRC$ but significantly higher prevalence of BHR than subjects without such a family history. There was no relation between cord serum IgE level and bronchial responsiveness. These results suggested that children with a genetic predisposition to develop asthma are at increased risk of having

BHR but not of having lower levels of lung function shortly after birth and before they developed any symptoms.

WHEEZING PHENOTYPES IN EARLY LIFE

The picture emerging from these data indicate the existence of a group of infants whose respiratory system may have a congenital form of limitation to airflow, and this developmental pattern becomes clinically important during infancy, that is, at a time when specific airflow conductance (i.e. the functional size of the airways relative to the size of the lungs) may be lower than that of older children. Infants belonging to this group are at increased risk of presenting with wheezing during viral respiratory infections, but they do not seem to have increased prevalence of BHR. The data suggest that this group of infants constitute the majority of subjects who wheeze in early life, and are more frequently represented among children with milder symptoms. Until recently, little was known, however, about the prognosis of these infants and about the factors associated with persistence of symptoms beyond the preschool years. In fact, many studies had suggested that most children with asthma start wheezing during infancy (Godfrey, 1984). Therefore, an important proportion of wheezing infants will go on to develop asthma, but it is not known if wheezing in infancy is the first manifestation of asthma in these children. The study by Tepper et al (1992) quoted earlier suggested that in subjects with a diagnosis of bronchiolitis, among whom hospitalization and thus more severe symptoms are more frequent, BHR is more prevalent than in control infants, and Young et al's (1991) data suggested that BHR may perhaps preexist bronchiolitis and be associated with a family history of asthma. The relation between this pre-disposition to asthma and the lower levels of lung function observed prior to any LRI (Martinez et al, 1991; Tager et al, 1993; Young et al, 1994) remained to be elucidated, but the results reported by Young et al also implied that a family history of asthma was not associated with lower $\dot{V}_{max}$FRC levels during the first months of life.

INFANT WHEEZING AND ALLERGIC SENSITIZATION

Allergic sensitization and higher IgE levels are significantly more common in schoolchildren with asthma than in children without this diagnosis (Burrows et al, 1989). The same does not hold true for wheezing in early life: there is now good evidence indicating that, as a group, children with a history of bronchiolitis or wheezing in infancy do not have increased IgE levels in cord blood (Halonen et al, 1992) nor are they more likely to be skin-test positive to aeroallergens later in life (Pullen and Hey, 1982). It is still possible, however, that a minority of wheezing infants whose symptoms may well be the first manifestation of asthma could coexist with the majority of infants who wheeze for mechanical reasons unrelated to an allergic inflammatory reaction occurring in the airways.

Data supporting this hypothesis was provided by Henderson et al (1992). These authors studied lung function and allergic sensitization in the group of 159 North Carolina school-age children whose history of wheezing episodes had been documented from early infancy and until age 6 by their paediatricians (Strope et al, 1991). As they had reported earlier, boys with two or more wheezing episodes during the first 6 years of life had lower levels of spirometric function. However, the authors now found that, in children with a history of recurrent wheezing in early life, increasingly more intense level of allergic sensitization to housedust mites (as assessed by radioimmunosorbent test, RAST) was correlated with progressively lower mean levels of small airway function. No such correlation was observed for boys without a history of recurrent wheezing in early life. It was not possible to determine from these data if prognosis of children with a history of recurrent wheezing in the first 6 years of life was modified by subsequent allergic sensitization. The authors speculated, however, that wheezing infants who subsequently were shown to be sensitized to house-dust mites may have been sensitized very early in life; that wheezing during infancy was 'associated' with this early sensitization; and that this association could explain the linkage between mite allergy and lower levels of lung function reported in their study. Henderson et al (1992) also found that mite sensitization was associated with increased BHR in both subjects with and without a history of recurrent wheezing in early life. The authors again speculated that only early mite sensitization was associated with lower levels of lung function, whereas both early and late sensitization would be associated with increased BHR.

Further evidence in favour of a possible role of early allergic sensitization to housedust mites in the development of early wheezing was provided by Sporik et al (1990). These authors found that the age of onset of wheez-ing in 11-year-old asthmatic children was inversely correlated with the concentration of housedust mites as measured in the children's homes around the age of 2 years. Sporik et al speculated that exposure to the antigens of housedust mites in early life was a risk factor for both early allergic sensitization and for early onset of asthmatic symptoms. However, because all subjects had a diagnosis of asthma by age 11, it was not possible to assess with this study the relation between the allergic sensitization and prognosis of wheezing in early life.

ASTHMA AND WHEEZING IN THE FIRST 6 YEARS OF LIFE

Our group recently reported the results of a longitudinal study of 826 children followed from birth and in whom most LRIs occurring during the first 3 years of life were ascertained by their paediatricians (Martinez et al, 1995). Serum IgE levels measured at a mean age of 9 months were available for most subjects, whereas results of pulmonary function tests ($\dot{V}_{max}$FRC) performed during infancy were available for 121 children. At a median age of 6 years, parents reported on wheezing episodes occurring during the previous year, and serum IgE levels, lung function tests, and skin-test reactivity to aeroallergens were also ascertained. Subjects were divided into four groups: those who had no wheezing LRIs during the first 3 years of life and who had no parental reports of wheezing episodes for the previous year at age 6 (never wheezers, 51%); those with one or more wheezing LRIs before age 3 but no current wheezing at age 6 (transient early wheezers, 20%); those with no wheezing LRIs in early life who had at least one episode of wheezing reported for the previous year at age 6 (late onset wheezers, 15%); and those who had one or more wheezing LRIs before age 3 and who were current wheezers at age 6 (persistent wheezers, 14%). It is important to stress that in this study, wheezing was ascertained in most cases at physical examination by the physician during the first 3 years of life, whereas parental reports were used to assess wheezing status at age 6. This discrepancy is almost inevitable: parents are much more likely to take their infant or toddler to the paediatrician for their wheezing than they are to take school-age children to the paediatrician for the same reason. Nevertheless, it is unlikely that biases in parental reporting at age 6 may explain the findings.

A first important feature is the very high cumulative incidence of wheezing episodes in this age group: by age 3, one third of all children had at least one wheezing LRI, and almost half had one or more wheezing episodes by age 6. Of all infants who had at least one wheezing LRI in the first 3 years of life, almost 60% had no wheezing episodes during the previous year at age 6.

Transient early wheezers were not more likely to be males, to have a maternal or paternal history of asthma, or to have eczema during the first year of life than never wheezers. Their mean serum IgE levels measured at birth, at a mean age of 9 months, and at age 6 were also not significantly different from those of never wheezers, as was a prevalence of positive skin test reactivity to allergens at age 6. However, transient early wheezers had markedly and significantly reduced length-adjusted $\dot{V}_{max}FRC$ during the first year of life when compared to never wheezers, late onset wheezers, and persistent wheezers. Height-adjusted $\dot{V}_{max}FRC$ at age 6 was still significantly lower in transient early wheezers than in never wheezers, in spite of the fact that the former were not actively wheezing at that age.

Persistent wheezers, on the other hand, had lung function values assessed shortly after birth that were not significantly different from those of never wheezers. However, by age 6, they had $\dot{V}_{max}FRC$ levels that were markedly lower than those of never wheezers. Their serum IgE levels were not increased in cord blood, but were already higher than those of all other groups at a mean age of 9 months and also at 6 years, at which time they were also significantly more likely to have a positive skin test to aeroallergens. Almost two-thirds of persistent wheezers were males, and they were almost four times more likely to have an asthmatic parent than never wheezers, and twice as likely to have eczema during the first year of life. They also had more frequent wheezing symptoms than transient early wheezers and parents reported that they noticed wheezing apart from colds more often in infants who would later become persistent wheezers than in transient early wheezers.

These results thus suggested that, for the majority of wheezing infants, their illness is a transitory phenomenon associated with diminished lung function in early life. These infants with a good prognosis are not, as a group, more genetically predisposed to develop asthma or allergies than the general population and they usually run out of their symptoms by age 6, perhaps because of the relatively faster growth of their airways compared with their lungs. Persistent wheezers, on the other hand, have increased prevalence of the same risk factors that are characteristic of older children with asthma: they have high serum IgE levels already during the first year of life, increased prevalence of allergic sensitization as infants, are more likely to be males, and are genetically predisposed to develop asthma. All the evidence thus suggests that many of these infants have a form of very early onset asthma.

Three characteristics of persistent wheezers in our data merit attention. First, these infants are probably born with lung function parameters that are not significantly lower than those of never wheezers. By age 6, however, they have significant deficits in mean $\dot{V}_{max}FRC$ values. This deterioration in lung function may be similar to that observed by Henderson et al (1992) among children with a history of recurrent wheezing before age 6 and who were sensitized to housedust mites: chronic allergic inflammation of the airways may be responsible for these changes. Second, cord serum IgE levels were not increased in persistent wheezers, but by 9 months of age, serum IgE levels were significantly higher in this group compared to never wheezers. This suggests that early allergic sensitization may indeed have occurred in these infants and that this may be associated with a worse prognosis. Finally, persistent wheezers had apparently more frequent and more severe symptoms in early life. This may explain why subjects with a diagnosis of bronchiolitis (Tepper et al, 1992) or who are hospitalized for wheezing LRIs in infancy seem to have a worse prognosis and are often found to have higher prevalence of BHR than wheezing infants with milder symptoms: early onset asthma may be over represented in this group.

SUMMARY

There is now little doubt that at least two groups of wheezing infants, whose symptoms have very different pathogenesis and prognosis, coexist in early life. Respiratory noises among transient early wheezers are probably the result of enhanced airway obstruction by mucus and oedema caused by respiratory infections in infants with congenitally narrower airway passages. In these children, lung function tracks with age and therefore, their lung function remains persistently lower than that of infants with no history of wheeze, even after symptoms have subsided. A smaller group of wheezing infants have early onset asthma, and in these subjects the airways are genetically predisposed to respond to viral and allergic inflammation, as is the case for older children with asthma. If these infants become sensitized to aeroallergens, recurrent episodes of airway obstruction will persist beyond the early years of life, and BHR that does not subside after infancy and deterioration of lung function will ensue. Identifying infants who will go on to develop persistent wheezing, and determining if inhaled anti-inflammatory drugs (Bisgaard et al, 1990) or other therapeutic approaches (Holt, 1994) can block the seemingly irreversible process leading to chronic asthma, is perhaps the most important challenge in the prevention of this common and invalidating condition.

Acknowledgement

The author was funded by a Research Development Award for Minority Faculty (HL-03154–01) from the National Institutes of Health.

REFERENCES

Bisgaard H, Munck SL, Nielsen JP et al (1990) Inhaled budesonide for treatment of recurrent wheezing in early childhood. *Lancet* **336:** 649–651.

Boesen I (1953) Asthmatic bronchitis in children. Prognosis for 162 cases, observed 6–11 years. *Acta Paediatrica* **42:** 87–96.

Burrows B, Martinez FD & Halonen M (1989) Association of asthma with serum IgE levels and skin-test reactivity to allergens. *New England Journal of Medicine* **320:** 271–277.

Clarke JR, Reese A & Silverman M (1992) Bronchial responsiveness and lung function in infants with lower respiratory tract illness over the first six months of life. *Archives of Disease in Childhood* **67:** 1454–1458.

Godfrey S (1984) The wheezy infant. In Meadow R (ed.) *Recent Advances in Paediatrics* **7:** 137–153.

Gurwitz D, Mindorff C & Levison H (1981) Increased incidence of bronchial reactivity in children with a history of bronchiolitis. *Journal of Pediatrics* **98:** 551–555.

Halonen M, Stern D, Taussig LM et al (1992) The predictive relationship between serum IgE levels at birth and subsequent incidences of lower respiratory tract illnesses and eczema in infants. *American Review of Respiratory Disease* **146:** 866–870.

Henderson FW, Stewart PW, Burchinal MR et al (1992) Respiratory allergy and the relationship between early childhood lower respiratory illness and subsequent lung function. *American Review of Respiratory Disease* **145:** 283–290.

Holt PG (1994) A potential vaccine strategy for asthma and allied atopic diseases during early childhood. *Lancet* **344:** 456–458.

Martinez FD, Morgan WJ, Wright AL et al (1988) Diminished lung function as a predisposing factor for wheezing respiratory illness in infants. *New England Journal of Medicine* **319:** 1112–1117.

Martinez FD (1991) Sudden infant death syndrome and small airway occlusion: facts and a hypothesis. *Pediatrics* **87:** 190–198.

Martinez FD. (ed.) *Childhood Asthma and Other Wheezing Disorders.* London: Chapman and Hall. Viral infection in early life. In Silverman M (in press).

Martinez FD, Morgan WJ, Wright AL et al (1991) Initial airway function is a risk factor for recurrent wheezing respiratory illnesses during the first three years of life. *American Review of Respiratory Disease* **143:** 312–316.

Martinez FD, Wright AL, Taussig LM et al (1995) Asthma and wheezing during the first 6 years of life. *New England Journal of Medicine* **332:** 133–138.

Mok JYQ & Simpson H (1982) Outcome of acute lower respiratory tract infections in infants: preliminary report of seven year follow-up study. *British Medical Journal* **285:** 333–337.

Morgan WJ (1990) Viral respiratory infection in infancy: provocation or propagation? *Seminars in Respiratory Medicine* **11:** 306–313.

Prendiville A, Green S & Silverman M (1987) Airway responsiveness in wheezy infants: evidence for functional beta adrenergic receptors. *Thorax* **42:** 100–104.

Pullen CR & Hey EN (1982) Wheezing, asthma, and pulmonary dysfunction 10 years after infection with respiratory syncytial virus in infancy. *British Medical Journal* **84:** 1665–1669.

Samet JM, Tager IB & Speizer FE (1983) The relationship between respiratory illness in childhood and chronic air-flow obstruction in adulthood. *American Review of Respiratory Disease* **127**: 508–523.

Sims DG, Downham MAPS, Gardner PS et al (1978) Study of 8 year old children with a history of respiratory syncytial virus bronchiolitis in infancy. *British Medical Journal* **1**: 11–14.

Sims DG, Gardner PS, Weightman D et al (1981) Atopy does not predispose to RSV bronchiolitis or postbronchiolitic wheezing. *British Medical Journal* **282**: 2086–2088.

Sporik R, Holgate ST, Platts-Mills TAE et al (1990) Exposure to house-dust mite allergen (Der p 1) and the development of childhood asthma: a prospective study. *New England Journal of Medicine* **323**: 502–507.

Stick SM, Arnott J, Turner DJ et al (1991) Bronchial responsiveness and lung function in recurrent wheezy infants. *American Review of Respiratory Disease* **144**: 1012–1015.

Strope GL, Stewart PW, Henderson FW et al (1991) Lung function in school-age children who had mild lower respiratory illnesses in early childhood. *American Review of Respiratory Disease* **144**: 655–662.

Tager IB, Hanrahan JP, Tosteson TD et al (1993) Lung function, prenatal and postnatal smoke exposure, and wheezing in the first year of life. *American Review of Respiratory Disease* **147**: 811–817.

Taussig LM, Landau LI, Godfrey S et al (1982) Determinants of forced expiratory flows in newborn infants. *Journal of Applied Physiology* **53**: 1220–1227.

Tepper RS, Rosenberg D & Eigen H (1992) Airway responsiveness in infants following bronchiolitis. *Pediatric Pulmonology* **13**: 6–10.

Voter KZ, Henry MM, Stewart PW et al (1988) Lower respiratory illness in early childhood and lung function and bronchial reactivity in adolescent males. *American Review of Respiratory Disease* **137**: 302–307.

Wilson NM, Phagoo SB & Silverman M (1992) Atopy, bronchial responsiveness and symptoms in wheezy 3-year olds. *Archives of Disease in Childhood* **67**: 491–495.

Wright AL, Taussig LM, Ray CG et al (1989) The Tucson Children's Respiratory Study. II. Lower respiratory tract illnesses in the first year of life. *American Journal of Epidemiology* **129**: 1232–1246.

Young S, Le Souef PN, Geelhoed GC et al (1991) Influence of a family history of asthma and parental smoking on airway responsiveness in early infancy. *New England Journal of Medicine* **324**: 1168–1173.

Young S, Arnott J, Le Souef PN et al (1994) Flow limitation during tidal expiration in symptom-free infants and the subsequent development of asthma. *Journal of Pediatrics* **124**: 681–688.

5

Asthma: classification, clinical patterns and natural history

PETER D. PHELAN
ANTHONY OLINSKY
HELMUT OSWALD

Asthma in children and adolescents is a very variable disorder. It has even been questioned as to whether it is essentially one disorder or a whole variety of different pathological processes that result in a common feature which is airways obstruction that varies from time to time either spontaneously or as a result of therapy. Many terms have been used to define patterns of childhood asthma—infection-induced asthma, allergen-induced asthma, exercise-induced asthma, steroid-resistant asthma. The general consensus is that there is a basic immunological disorder which results in inflammation of the airways mucosa and a variable degree of bronchial muscle spasm.

In this chapter it will be assumed that there is basically one disorder called asthma but it covers a wide spectrum: from a child in the first 4–6 years of life who has a number of episodes of wheeze and cough triggered by intercurrent viral infections, to an adolescent whose only symptom is wheeze during exercise, to the patient who has daily or near daily symptoms as a result of longstanding airways obstruction.

The single most important feature in the management of asthma is to define its severity. If this is not done, then treatment will be inappropriate. There are data which indicate that children in whom asthma is a relatively trivial problem are overtreated whereas many of those in whom it is having a major impact on lifestyle continue to be underrecognized and consequently undertreated (Jones et al, 1987; Hill et al, 1989). In the characterization of the severity of asthma it is important to define the severity of acute symptoms, and for long-term management it is important to define the impact the asthma has on lifestyle. To do that it is necessary to estimate the frequency of acute episodes and the frequency and severity of interval symptoms.

There is now much information on the natural history of childhood asthma into adult life. However, for this to be helpful in the management of individual patients and in counselling families, it needs to be related to the clinical patterns in childhood.

Baillière's Clinical Paediatrics—
Vol. 3, No. 2, May 1995
ISBN 0–7020–1986–0

CLASSIFICATION OF ACUTE EPISODES OF ASTHMA

There is a spectrum in severity of acute episodes of asthma from one in which there is some cough, audible wheeze but little or no respiratory distress, to those that rapidly progress to respiratory failure with a high risk of death if appropriate treatment is not rapidly instituted. Any classification will be arbitrary and one group will merge into the other (Bishop et al, 1992). However, there is some value in adopting a classification system that relates to the appropriate level of therapy.

Mild acute episodes

These are characterized by wheeze, perhaps some cough with little or no respiratory distress. They are commonly triggered by intercurrent viral infection, exercise, laughing and occasionally exposure to allergens. The patient is well oxygenated in air, there is little or no elevation in the respiratory rate and the child or adolescent is able to say five, six or more words between breaths. There is no use of accessory muscles of respiration and lower rib recession during inspiration is minimal.

These episodes may last for a few minutes as after exercise or 24–48 hours if they are triggered by a viral infection. In such circumstances, sleep is not disturbed.

Moderate acute episodes

With a moderate acute episode of asthma, there is both subjective and objective evidence of respiratory distress. Cough and wheeze again remain the dominant symptoms but, if old enough, the patient may complain of breathlessness. In general the child or adolescent may prefer to sit or lie down. There will be no cyanosis but the respiratory rate will be increased and there will be a need to take a breath after every three to five words. In younger children particularly with a more compliant ribcage, there is likely to be lower rib recession during inspiration and as a consequence, to maintain adequate inspiratory changes in lung volume, some use of accessory muscles of respiration. Therefore the upper chest will expand during inspiration while there may be a decrease in circumference in the lower chest giving parodoxical movement. Breath sounds in the chest on auscultation will not be diminished and there will be widespread inspiratory and expiratory wheezes.

A severe, acute episode of asthma

With a severe episode of asthma, there is impairment of gas exchange and a risk of respiratory failure. The patient will be cyanosed in air and respiration will be heaving with marked use of accessory muscles and again lower rib recession. There is likely to be an audible wheeze but with progressive increase in the degree of airways obstruction, tidal volume is likely to fall and wheeze may become relatively soft despite increased inspiratory and expiratory effort. There will be a marked increase in respiratory rate and the patient may have difficulty in saying more than one or two words between breaths. Breath sounds may be decreased on auscultation and again depending on the tidal volume, inspiratory and expiratory wheezes heard in the chest.

As a severe episode progresses, there is likely to be further reduction in tidal volume and if diaphragmatic failure intervenes, then a reduction in minute volume. Wheeze may then become very soft or even absent, breath sounds markedly reduced and few wheezes may be heard in the chest. Such a patient is in grave risk of death if medical intervention does not immediately occur.

LONG-TERM PATTERN

With the widespread availability of effective prophylactic drugs, the long-term classification of asthma has assumed increasing importance. While it is now recognized that prophylactic drugs almost certainly do not alter the long-term course of asthma, they can have a substantial impact on morbidity. Some of them are not free of side effects and therefore their benefit must outweigh their risks.

The long-term pattern of asthma can be best characterized in terms of its impact on the child and family's lifestyle and in those over the age of 6–7 years, the presence of abnormal lung function between acute episodes.

The use of terms to define the long-term pattern of asthma is most important. Names such as chronic asthma or severe asthma in relation to long-term create great confusion in the minds of health care providers and patients. Two episodes a year over 4–5 years may suggest to some that the asthma is a chronic disease and this is true. Similarly, one or two severe acute episodes may make parents believe their child has severe asthma. It is much better to classify the long-term pattern of asthma in terms of the frequency of acute attacks and the presence or absence of interval symptoms between those attacks (Rosier et al, 1994). This relates much better to morbidity. While in general the less frequent the acute episodes, the less severe they are, there are frequent exceptions.

Again, the three patterns suggested are arbitrary and one merges into the other. However, these have been shown to be helpful in predicting the long-term course of asthma (Oswald et al, 1994) and in determining the need for appropriate prophylactic therapy.

Infrequent episodic asthma

At least 75% of children with asthma fall into this pattern (McNicol and Williams, 1973). It is simply defined as acute episodes of asthma occurring less frequently than every 4–6 weeks with minimal or no interval symptoms. If interval symptoms do occur they are almost always exercise-induced and often quite prolonged exercise, e.g. running 400 m or more is required before any wheeze or breathing difficulty occurs.

In general the acute episodes tend to be either mild or less often moderate, but there is the occasional child, particularly in the preschool and early school years who may have two or three severe episodes of asthma a year without interval symptoms. Between the episodes, lung function, in particular spirometry, is normal. Other allergic features are usually not particularly prominent.

As is discussed in Chapter 4, when such episodes occur in the first 2–3 years of life, it can be impossible to tell whether they are purely viral infection-induced wheeze or a manifestation of asthma. It is probably only about a third of minor wheezing episodes in the first 3 years of life that are genuinely a manifestation of asthma.

Frequent episodic asthma

Once episodes of wheeze lasting 12–48 hours are occurring more frequently than every 4–6 weeks, they are beginning to have a significant impact on a child's or adolescent's lifestyle. Again, should interval symptoms occur they are most frequently induced by exercise. In this group perhaps less exercise will be necessary to produce breathing discomfort and wheeze than in those with infrequent episodic asthma. This pattern is present in about 20% of children with asthma.

In general children and adolescents in this group tend to have acute episodes of a moderate degree of severity although there can be considerable variation in severity from episode to episode. Between the episodes, lung function should be normal or at most there should be some minor reduction in FEV_1 and FEF_{25-75} (Hill et al, 1972). This should be completely reversed with one dose of a β_2 sympathomimetic.

Other allergic features such as hay fever, eczema or a history of urticaria are more common in this group than in those with infrequent episodic asthma. Episodes in these children may be triggered by intercurrent viral infection, exposure to allergen, or weather change although for the great majority no trigger factor can be predicted. In general the episodes last for some days and during these the child's level of activity is often reduced.

Persistent asthma

The pattern of frequent episodic asthma gradually merges into persistent asthma and the separation relates to the frequency and severity of interval symptoms. By the time the child or adolescent is having symptoms of wheeze requiring the immediate use of a β_2 sympathomimetic more frequently than once or twice a week, it is reasonable to assume that they have ongoing airways obstruction. The more troublesome the persistent asthma the more frequent the interval symptoms and in general the more severe the acute exacerbations.

Characteristic of more troublesome persistent asthma is waking during the night with wheeze or chest tightness requiring the use of a β_2 sympathomimetic, chest tightness and wheeze when first awakening in the morning and symptomatic bronchoconstriction readily induced by relatively minor exercise. About 5% of children with asthma have this pattern and the majority of those affected in childhood and early adolescence are males although by mid-adolescence there is no longer a gender difference. The reasons for this are not known.

Children and adolescents with more troublesome persistent asthma will often have a chest wall deformity either a barrel chest or pigeon chest with Harrison's sulci. There will frequently be wheezes in the chest while the patient says it is an average day or they will be readily induced by coughing and forced expiration.

At the mild end of persistent asthma FEV_1 may be normal or near normal although the shape of a flow volume curve will generally show concavity towards the x axis and reduced FEF_{25-75} (Hill et al, 1972). Peak expiratory flow rate will not pick up these minor degrees of airways obstruction. At the other end of the spectrum is the child or adolescent with severe airways obstruction which does not improve following a single dose of β_2 agonist. Often a course of oral corticosteroids is necessary to demonstrate bronchodilator responsiveness in this group.

The lifestyle of these children and their families can be seriously impaired by their asthma. There are frequent disturbed nights, substantial amounts of time are missed from school and the child or adolescent's ability to participate in sport is seriously impaired.

UNUSUAL PATTERN OF ASTHMA

Persistent wheeze in the first year of life

There are some infants who develop, during the early months of life, a pattern of persistent wheeze that is present most days particularly when the child is active or excited. There may be little disturbance in the child's well-being and level of activity by quite a loud wheeze. These children grow and develop normally. From time to time, particularly with intercurrent infections, the wheeze may produce some degree of breathing distress. The relationship of this pattern of wheeze to asthma is not clear as there have not been adequate long-term studies. It is uncommon for these infants to have eczema or other evidence of an atopic background.

Bronchodilators are ineffective and the severity of the symptoms should not justify the use of prophylactic drugs. Further, they do not seem to alter the pattern of wheeze.

Whether wheeze is the result of abnormally small airways or alternatively a manifestation of asthma will only be resolved by proper long-term study. The most important aspect in recognizing this pattern is to ensure that these infants are not overtreated.

Hyper-secretory asthma

There seem to be children, particularly in the toddler and early school years, whose acute episodes of asthma are characterized by the production of large amounts of mucus. This may result in quite extensive areas of segmental or even lobar collapse. An occasional older child or adolescent can develop a total lung collapse again presumably due to excess secretion of mucus.

It is important that the role of mucus in causing a segmental, lobar or lung collapse is recognized. The essential treatment for these episodes is bronchodilators and perhaps corticosteroids. If the collapse is prolonged there may be a risk of secondary bacterial infection but antibiotics are not required during the acute episodes.

Cough variant asthma

Currently in a number of countries there seems to be much overdiagnosis of asthma in children whose sole symptom is recurrent episodes of cough lasting some days to 6–8 weeks. In these children, cough may initially be loose and rattly but more typically is hard and dry. It may be perceived by the family as being worse at night. However, objective measures of cough in children have demonstrated there is often a poor correlation between parental report both of periodicity, frequency and severity and objective measurement (Archer and Simpson, 1985). One family may accept a pattern of cough in a child as normal whereas a similar pattern in a different family with a greater level of anxiety or different life experiences would give concern about serious underlying disease.

Epidemiological studies would suggest that somewhere between 10 and 20% of children have repeated periods of quite prolonged cough (Clifford et al, 1989). There is almost no evidence to support existence of a disorder of 'cough variant asthma' in which cough is the sole symptom. There should be great reluctance in diagnosing asthma in a child with no evidence of airways obstruction such as audible wheeze, wheezes on auscultation of the chest or some evidence of impaired airways function.

Most likely these children with repeated episodes of quite prolonged cough have a cough induced by viral infection. Postnasal drip and sinusitis do not cause cough in children although persistent nasal obstruction may result in bronchial irritation because of the inhalation of nonhumidified air by the child who cannot breathe through his or her nose.

THE NATURAL HISTORY OF CHILDHOOD ASTHMA

Knowledge of the natural history of childhood asthma is essential if the long-term benefits of therapy are to be properly evaluated and patients and families appropriately counselled.

There are a number of studies that have followed children with asthma through childhood and adolescence into adult life (Blair, 1977; Martin et al, 1980; Gerritsen et al, 1989; Jenkins et al, 1994). However, most of them have not been randomly selected community based, a number have seen children on only two occasions and few have characterized the severity of the asthma through childhood. The Melbourne epidemiological study of childhood asthma has followed children with wheeze from the age of 7 through to the age of 35 and much of this section will be based on the findings of that study (Oswald et al, 1994). However, it had a number of significant deficiencies in that the control group was too small to allow any assessment of the risk of developing asthma subsequent to the age of 7. Furthermore, the history at age 7 was retrospective and parents may well have forgotten a few minor episodes of wheeze in the early years of life. The age at which the wheezing episodes had occurred prior to 7 was not specifically recorded.

More recent studies have helped to correct some of these deficiencies. The work of Martinez and his colleagues in Tucson as documented in Chapter 4 of this book clarifies many of the issues related to wheezing in the early years of life. Their studies would suggest that approximately one in three children who have wheeze prior to the age of 2–3 years with inter-current viral infection continue to wheeze in later childhood. In the Melbourne study children classified as mild wheezy bronchitis at the age of 7 (Williams and McNicol, 1969) and who would fall into the clinical pattern of infrequent episodic asthma probably comprised some children who had wheeze purely due to viral infection and others in whom the wheeze occurred because of asthma.

In Figure 1 is shown the cumulative age of the first episode of wheezing in children who develop asthma before the age of 16 years. This has been constructed from community based studies (Williams and McNicol, 1969; Zeidan et al, 1988) and in these the current hypothesis of two different causes of wheeze in the first 2–3 years of life was not clearly identified. Therefore it may over-emphasise the number of children with asthma whose wheeze commences prior to the age of 3. Nevertheless the data do suggest that about 50% of children with asthma will have had their first wheezy episode before the age of 3–4 years, 80% before the age of 7 and a further 20% develop it between the ages of 7 and 16 years.

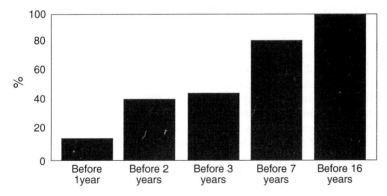

Figure 1. Cumulative age of onset of asthma in childhood and early adolescence.

A much higher percentage of children with persistent asthma have their first episode of wheeze prior to the age of 12 months than those with infrequent episodic asthma. However, even allowing for the fact that perhaps two-thirds of infants with wheeze in the first 2–3 years of life will not have asthma, the majority of those who do wheeze as a result of asthma in the first year of life are likely to have infrequent episodic asthma because it is much more common than persistent asthma.

If the first episode of wheeze is after the age of 3 years, then the child is more likely to have less troublesome asthma and fall into the patterns of either infrequent or frequent episodic asthma.

The course of asthma in the three arbitrarily defined clinical groups will now be discussed based predominantly on the Melbourne epidemiological study. However, in general the other epidemiological studies support these findings.

Infrequent episodic asthma

Over half the children with this pattern of asthma have their first episode of wheeze after the age of 3 years. Most of the episodes in the early years of life seem to be triggered by intercurrent viral infection and are relatively mild. They are most frequent in the preschool and early school years when the frequency of viral infection in all children is at a maximum. After the age of 6 or 7 years, some episodes may occur without an obvious trigger but parents attribute some of these to weather change or exposure to allergens. In later childhood and adolescence, patients who have had this pattern of asthma may notice some exercise-induced wheeze after prolonged running. However, this is rarely troublesome.

Forty to 50% of children with this pattern of wheeze have ceased to have episodes by the age of 10 years although a few may continue to have minor exercise symptoms without clearly recognizing these as asthma. In another 10–20% the episodes resolve during adolescence. By early to mid adult life fewer than 40% of these subjects continue to have any asthma symptoms. However, perhaps 10–20% whose asthma had apparently resolved by the end of the first decade have some recurrence of symptoms during adolescence or early adult life and occasionally these can be quite troublesome. Because the history of symptoms during childhood and early adolescence are normally taken from parents and from the subject themselves in late adolescence and adult life, parents may not have been aware of mild symptoms in later childhood and early adolescence so there may never have been true clearing. However, if the subject who has recurrence of wheezing in adult life was not aware of their childhood history, such recurrence could well be labelled as adult onset asthma.

In the majority of those who had a pattern of infrequent episode asthma and who continue to have symptoms into adult life, the wheeze is minor and occurs mainly with exercise and intercurrent respiratory infection (Figure 2). Many would not consider themselves as having asthma. Very few develop persistent asthma as adults.

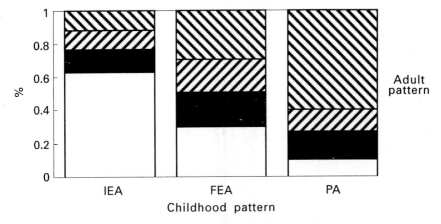

Figure 2. Pattern of asthma in adult life in relation to that in childhood. □, ceased; ■, IEA; □, FEA; □, PA.

Lung function in this group of subjects is normal throughout childhood and adolescence and into adult life (Figure 3). Bronchial reactivity in adult life in those whose asthma has resolved is no different from a control group and even in those with occasional mild symptoms (Kelly et al, 1988), it is normal.

The presence or absence of allergy at age 7 years is not predictive of whether wheeze would continue or not (Oswald et al, 1994). There seems to be no way of identifying those whose wheezing episodes will resolve completely and those who will continue to have minor symptoms as adults.

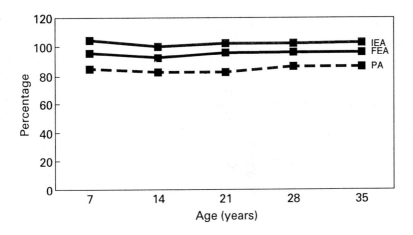

Figure 3. FEV₁ (% predicted) at 7, 14, 21, 28 and 35 years in those who had IEA, FEA and PA in childhood.

Frequent episodic asthma

Almost three-quaters of children with frequent episodic asthma will have had their initial episode of wheeze prior to the age of 3 years. They continue to have episodes of wheeze throughout childhood and adolescence. In the early years of life most episodes seem to be triggered by viral infection but by the age of 7 or 8 years, episodes are occurring without obvious cause.

Allergen exposure presumably is an important factor in some episodes and again parents often comment on weather change as being important. Wheezing is relatively easily brought on by exercise but will usually be prevented by prior inhalation of a β_2 sympathomimetic.

The episodes seem to be most frequent and most troublesome between the ages of 7 and 12 years, and often during adolescence their frequency and severity progressively decreases. However, only about 25% of these subjects lose all their asthma symptoms by early adult life and continue to be wheeze-free into their mid thirties (Figure 2). About 20% of those with continuing symptoms have them quite infrequently. In about half the remainder the asthma seems to become more troublesome in early adult life and there are now interval symptoms. Girls in general seem to be more likely to develop persistent symptoms than boys.

In this group there is minor impairment of lung function between the episodes throughout childhood and adolescence and it is only in those adults in whom the asthma has become persistent is there evidence of significant airways obstruction.

Persistent asthma

Early onset of symptoms is characteristic of the child who will have persistent asthma during childhood, adolescence and into adult life. A quarter will have commenced wheezing prior to the age of 6 months and three-quarters by the age of 3 years. Many have periods of quite prolonged wheezing in the first 1 to 2 years of life.

The asthma seems to be most troublesome between the ages of 8 and 14 years. Airways obstruction will often be present for months at a time. Many of these children are never totally wheeze-free. They wake two to three nights a week with symptoms of asthma requiring a bronchodilator. They frequently have chest tightness when they first awaken in the morning. Their physical activities are limited by easily induced airways obstruction which is only partially prevented by the prior use of a β_2 sympathomimetic. In the more severely affected patients, growth is retarded more so in weight than height and puberty is delayed.

As already mentioned 80% of those with this pattern of asthma in childhood are male. However, during puberty boys seem to improve more than girls. Why there should be this gender difference is unknown. Only about 5% of children with this pattern of asthma will become wheeze-free as adults. Sixty percent will continue to have persistent asthma characterized by acute episodes and interval symptoms. In the remaining 40% the asthma seems less troublesome in adult life than it was during childhood and adolescence. In only about 10% does it become a trivial complaint.

The subjects continue to show airways obstruction throughout childhood, adolescence and into adult life. In many this is severe. However, by 35 almost none have developed irreversible airways disease. However, it seems probable that in some this will occur by later adult life.

Subjects with persistent asthma will often have troublesome allergic features. Almost all have hay fever and many were troubled by eczema in childhood and this continues into adult life.

SUMMARY

Asthma is probably the commonest cause of chronic ill health among children yet its management continues to be unsatisfactory. The major reason for this is the failure to define acute episodes in terms of their degree of respiratory distress and its long-term pattern in terms of the frequency of acute episodes and the presence or otherwise of interval symptoms between those. Acute episodes should be characterized in terms of mild, moderate and severe and the long-term pattern in terms of infrequent episodes, frequent episodes and persistent asthma. This then allows appropriate consideration for the natural history of the disorder and is the basis for therapeutic decisions. Fifty to 60% of children with the pattern of infrequent episodic asthma will be wheeze-free as adults whereas only 25% of those with frequent episodes apparently are asthma-free as adults. Ninety to 95% of those with persistent asthma in childhood will continue to have asthma as adults and in at least half of these it remains troublesome.

REFERENCES

Archer LNJ & Simpson H (1985) Night cough counts and diary card scores in asthma. *Archives of Diseases in Childhood* **60:** 473–474.
Bishop J, Carlin J & Nolan TM (1992) Evaluation of the properties and reliability of a clinical severity scale for acute asthma in children. *Journal of Clinical Epidemiology* **45:** 71–76.
Blair H (1977) Natural history of childhood asthma. *Archives of Diseases in Childhood* **52:** 613–618.
Clifford RD, Radford M, Howell JB et al (1989) Prevalence of respiratory symptoms among 7 and 11 year old schoolchildren and association with asthma. *Archives of Diseases in Childhood* **64:** 1118–1125.
Gerritsen J, Koeter H, Postma S et al (1989) Prognosis of asthma from childhood to adulthood. *American Review of Respiratory Disease* **140:** 1325–1330.
Hill RA, Standen PJ & Tattersfield AE (1989) Asthma, wheezing, and school absence in primary schools. *Archives of Diseases in Childhood* **64:** 246–251.
Hill DJ, Landau LI, McNicol, KN et al (1972) Asthma—the physiological and clinical spectrum in childhood. *Archives of Diseases in Childhood* **47:** 874–881.
Jones DT, Sears MR, Holdaway MD et al (1987) Childhood asthma in New Zealand. *British Journal of Diseases of the Chest* **81:** 332–340.
Jenkins MA, Hopper JL, Bowes G et al (1994) Factors in childhood as predictors of asthma in adult life. *British Medical Journal* **309:** 90–93.
Kelly W, Hudson I, Raven J et al (1988) Childhood asthma and adult lung function. *American Review of Respiratory Diseases* **138:** 26–30.

McNicol KN & Williams HE (1973) Spectrum of asthma in children—I, Clinical and physiological components. *British Medical Journal* **4:** 7–11.

Martin AJ, McLennan LA, Landau LI et al (1980) The natural history of childhood asthma to adult life. *British Medical Journal* **280:** 1397–1400.

Oswald H, Phelan PD, Lanigan A et al (1994) Outcome of childhood asthma in midadult life. *British Medical Journal* **309:** 95–96.

Rosier MJ, Bishop J, Nolan T et al (1994) Measurement of functional severity of asthma in children. *American Journal of Respiratory and Critical Care Medicine* **149:** 1434–1441.

Williams H & McNicol KN (1969) Prevalence, natural history and relationship to wheezy bronchitis and asthma in children. An epidemiological study. *British Medical Journal* **4:** 321–325.

Zeidan S, Ali H, Danskin MJ et al (1988) The temporal pattern and natural history of asthma in childhood. *Archives of Diseases in Children* **63:** 697.

6

Pathophysiology and lung function tests in the assessment and management of childhood asthma

R. G. GARY RUIZ
JOHN F. PRICE

Lung function tests enable objective assessment of asthmatic children. Age and ability will often limit the use that can be made of standard tests. When they are possible measurements can be invaluable in directing appropriate clinical management. This chapter focuses on tests which may be used in routine practice rather than in research. It is divided into three sections. The first describes the mechanics of breathing and how they are disturbed by asthma, as it is these disturbances which are reflected by lung function tests. The next section deals with the tests themselves, how they are performed, what they measure and their pitfalls. Finally there is a discussion on the role these tests may have in the management of asthma in children.

PHYSIOLOGY AND PATHOPHYSIOLOGY

A résumé of how normal breathing occurs and a definition of lung volumes and capacities is given. This is followed by a description of the mechanics of forced expiration because it not only helps to explain asthma pathophysiology but the rationale of the most useful tests of lung function (West, 1987).

Mechanics of breathing

The aim of breathing is to move air into and out of the alveoli to permit gas exchange with pulmonary arterial blood by diffusion across the alveolar–capillary interface. Inspiration is achieved by lowering alveolar pressure to below atmospheric pressure. This occurs when the diaphragm contracts depressing abdominal contents and raising the rib cage thereby increasing intrathoracic volume. Rather like inflating a balloon, a recoil pressure is generated by inflating the lungs. Normal quiet expiration is produced by this elastic recoil pressure and is thus passive.

Only when the whole lung is collapsed such as with a pneumothorax will the recoil pressure become zero. The chest wall also exerts a recoil pressure tending to spring it outwards and therefore in the opposite direction to lung recoil. Normal quiet expiration ends when the inward lung recoil balances the outward chest wall recoil. The lung volume at this point is the functional residual capacity or FRC (see below). Chest wall recoil is minimal during infancy and increases with age.

When panting during exercise, coughing or breathing against airway obstruction a pressure greater than the lung recoil is required. Expiration then becomes active and may continue below FRC. This is achieved by contraction of abdominal muscles which push the diaphragm up and possibly the internal intercostal muscles which depress the rib cage. The changes in pulmonary dynamics which occur when pressure in addition to just passive lung recoil is employed to bring about expiration, are best appreciated after considering the extreme case of a forced expiration. It would be helpful to review the standard divisions of lung volume beforehand.

Lung volumes and capacities

There are four primary lung volumes. Tidal volume (V_T) is the volume inspired and expired with each normal quiet breath. Residual volume (RV) is the volume remaining in the lungs after a maximal expiration. Inspiratory reserve volume (IRV) is the maximum volume which can be inhaled above a tidal inspiration. Expiratory reserve volume (ERV) is the maximum volume which can be exhaled after a tidal expiration. Direct spirometry measures volumes of air moving in and out of the lungs directly. All the volumes can be determined in this way apart from RV.

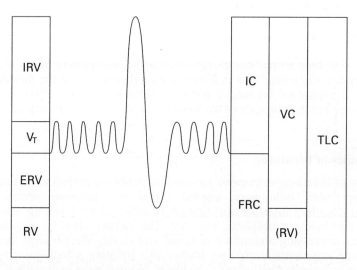

Figure 1. Spirogram showing the four lung volumes and the four lung capacities. (See text for explanation of the abbreviations.)

Lung capacities consist of two or more lung volumes as shown in Figure 1. There are four lung capacities: functional residual capacity (FRC), vital capacity (VC), total lung capacity (TLC) and inspiratory capacity (IC). VC and IC can be obtained by direct spirometry.

This leaves FRC, TLC and RV which cannot be measured directly. In practice only FRC needs to be measured by indirect spirometry (gas dilution or body plethysmography) as RV and TLC can then be derived from a knowledge of the direct measurements (Figure 1).

Mechanics of forced expiration

During forced expiration the accessory muscles of respiration are used to generate a positive intra-pleural pressure which is transmitted to the alveoli increasing the pressure driving air out of the lung. This is analogous to squirting air out of a syringe: the greater the force applied the faster the flow out of the syringe. However, unlike this model, the airways are within the thorax so that the propelling force is not simply applied to one end of the airways but transmitted to their length as well, tending to compress them.

Consider the pressures in various parts of the lung during maximal forced expiration from TLC (Figure 2). Normally intrapleural pressure (P_{pl}) is negative but during forced expiration the expiratory muscles generate a very positive P_{pl}. The pressure in the alveolus, P_A, is equal to the lung recoil (P_L) plus P_{pl}. Air flow out of the lung occurs because of the pressure drop from P_A to atmospheric pressure at the mouth (P_{atm}). At some point along the airway the pressure within P_{aw} will fall to the pressure outside P_{pl}. This is called the equal pressure point (EPP). Downstream (away from the alveolus) to the EPP, intrapleural pressure causes dynamic compression of the airway tending to close it.

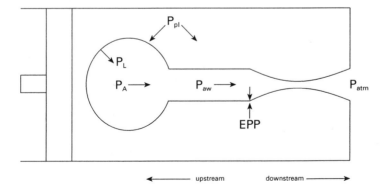

Figure 2. Schematic representation of alveolar airspace connected to an airway leading to the mouth enclosed within the chest with an expanded intrapleural space. The muscles of expiration are represented by a piston. (See text for explanation of the abbreviations.)

The important point to note is that flow out of the alveolus can only be increased by increasing effort until dynamic compression occurs. Thereafter increasing the driving pressure simply compresses the airway more so that there is no increase in flow. In other words flow is affected by resistance of the upstream segment but becomes independent of effort.

Consider flow in the upstream segment in isolation. Flow in a tube is proportional to the pressure drop and to the resistance (which is dependent on the diameter). The EPP must occur where the alveolar pressure has fallen by an amount equal to the lung recoil (as $P_A = P_{pl} + P_L$). The pressure drop is therefore the lung recoil pressure. During the effort-independent phase of forced expiration, flow is dependent on lung recoil pressure and resistance of the upstream segment.

The position of the EPP is affected by the lung volume because lung recoil falls as the lung deflates. It will move upstream as forced expiration progresses. Only the smaller airways remain upstream towards the end of a forced expiration and determine flow. Increased resistance of the upstream segment would also move the EPP upstream as the pressure drop would occur sooner.

Although we have described the pulmonary dynamics during a forced expiration some of the same mechanisms operate even with normal breathing. Intra-thoracic pressures vary between regions of the lung. When upright, intrapleural pressure is higher at the bases due to gravity and may even be positive. At low lung volumes (approaching RV) this may be sufficient to cause dynamic closure of basal airways. The lung volume at which this starts to occur is called the 'closing capacity'. The difference between RV and closing capacity is the closing volume.

Pathophysiology of asthma

Asthma is manifested by widespread airways obstruction. This may occur by three mechanisms: mucus plugging within the airway lumen; swelling of the respiratory epithelium lining the wall; and bronchoconstriction. Lung mechanics can be reviewed in the light of increased resistance produced by narrowing of the airways.

Asthma may be regarded as a disease mainly of expiration until it becomes severe. Inspiration tends to expand the airways as well as air spaces reducing resistance to flow. Expiration, however, has the opposite effect of compressing airways exacerbating air flow obstruction. Dynamic airways compression, of course, limits how far air flow can be maintained in the face of higher resistance by increasing expiratory effort. Measures of expiratory flow are therefore reduced in asthma.

As previously explained, airway narrowing moves the EPP upstream. This means that dynamic compression occurs earlier in expiration at higher lung volume. Not only does this occur during a forced breath but during quiet expiration basal airways will close prematurely as well. This produces an increase in RV (and therefore FRC) by air trapping (Figure 3). Having to breathe at higher lung volumes increases the work of breathing and causes dyspnoea. Increased RV encroaches on the vital capacity which therefore decreases. The fall in vital capacity does not usually avert an overall increase in total lung capacity caused by higher FRC (Blackie et al, 1990). Thus hyperinflation may be regarded as an indication of small airways obstruction.

With increasing severity of an asthma attack, airway closure on expiration occurs at higher and higher lung volumes and the lungs may become considerably hyperinflated. This increases the elastic lung recoil and may reduce airway resistance by applying more radial traction. Expiration may then become easier than inspiration.

During an asthma attack there is widespread ventilation perfusion mismatching tending to cause hypoxaemia much more than hypercapnia. This stimulates peripheral chemoreceptors to increase alveolar ventilation which will often result in a low arterial PCO_2 initially. It is only after such severe airway obstruction that alveolar ventilation falls that PCO_2 begins to rise.

STANDARD TESTS OF LUNG FUNCTION

In childhood asthma standard tests of lung function used in clinical practice are of three types. The easiest to perform and most useful are the tests of forced expiration. Not only do they determine the presence of airways obstruction but measure the degree. Second is the measurement of static lung volumes and capacities. Finally there are the tests demonstrating

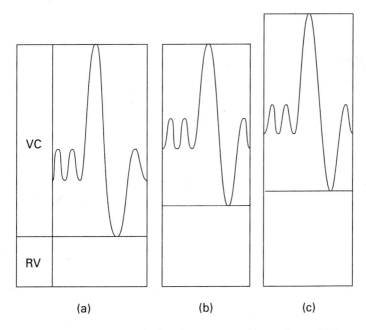

Figure 3. Lung volume changes occurring in asthma. (a) Normal lung volumes, (b) air trapping, (c) hyperinflation i.e. where TLC is increased. Note how RV and FRC increase and VC decreases.

bronchial hyperresponsiveness, a characteristic feature of asthma. Other tests such as the measurement of airway resistance or conductance, lung compliance, pulmonary gas distribution, etc, can be made in children but are mainly research tools, not used in routine practice and beyond the scope of this chapter.

Tests of forced expiration

Spirometry

Forced expiratory spirometry is probably the best standardized of all lung function tests. Spirometers measure the volumes of air inhaled and/or exhaled in relation to time. There are essentially two types, those which measure volume directly by collection or displacement and those which primarily measure flow. The former are more precise and used to establish spirometric standards. Some convert movement into an electrical signal which generates the spirogram introducing an extra calibration requirement.

Flow measuring spirometers calculate volume indirectly by electronically integrating flow with the time over which it occurs. They are more portable and more suited to frequent or continuous measurement but their accuracy is dependent on flow being laminar and they obviously require careful and frequent calibration.

With either type of spirometer, if flow and volume are converted to electric signals, they can be fed into an electronic recording system which can plot one against the other during a breathing manoeuvre generating a flow/volume curve in inspiration and expiration or a flow/volume loop.

Spirometers used for children should be accurate to ± 50 ml (Becklake et al, 1991). The volume measured in a spirometer is at ambient temperature and pressure and 100% saturated with water vapour (ATPS). Within the lungs, this volume would have been at body temperature (BTPS). For accurate volume determination measurements should be converted to BTPS conditions.

Forced expiratory volume and flow

In the forced vital capacity (FVC) manoeuvre the child inspires to TLC and exhales as rapidly as possible to RV. FVC is the total volume exhaled in the manoeuvre (Figure 4). It should be similar to the vital capacity measured on slow exhalation and the significance of its reduction in asthma has been described.

The volume exhaled in the first second is the forced expiratory volume in 1 second, FEV_1 (Figure 4). It is reduced in the presence of airways obstruction. Normal adults can usually exhale at least 70% of their vital capacity in the first second and the FEV_1/FVC ratio is sometimes used as an index of airways obstruction. This is not generally useful in children, however, because they can often reach FVC within 1 second of starting the manoeuvre. $FEV_{0.75}$ has been suggested as a more appropriate parameter for children (Cogswell et al, 1975) but has not been widely adopted.

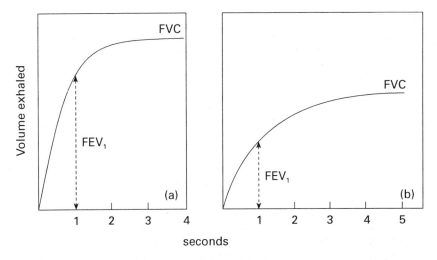

Figure 4. Volume/time curves obtained with a forced vital capacity manoeuvre on a spirometer (e.g. Vitalogram®) in (a) a normal child and (b) a similar size child with airways obstruction.

Early in a forced expiration, flow is driven by expiratory effort but it rapidly becomes effort-independent due to dynamic airways compression. The FEV_1 spans both periods and may therefore be a relatively effort-dependent parameter. Maximal FEV_1 is not actually achieved by maximal effort because it causes a greater compression of alveolar air space which reduces the initial lung volume (Krowka et al, 1987). It is important therefore to ensure maximal effort so that FEV_1 is not overestimated as well as underestimated.

Forced expiratory flow (FEF) rates can be averaged between different points in a forced expiration. $FEF_{25-75\%}$ averages flow over the middle 50% of the FVC and is given by the slope of the line connecting the points on the spirogram at 25 and 75% FVC. It is a more sensitive indicator of flow in the smaller bronchi and larger bronchioles than FEV_1 but is less reproducible (Hutchison et al, 1981) and particularly in children less useful for routine testing.

Maximum expiratory flow volume (MEFV) curve

The flow volume curve reveals further information from an FVC manoeuvre. We assume that when dynamic compression occurs, flow in the upstream segment determines the measured expiratory flow. At low lung volumes the equal pressure point moves into the small airways and measurements such as $FEF_{75\%}$ (maximal flow when 75% of the vital capacity has been exhaled) therefore reflect flow in the small airways. When there is limitation of flow at lower lung volumes, this part of the MEFV curve may have a scooped out appearance (Figure 5). This is more marked in emphysema, where the increased propensity towards dynamic airways compression is due to loss of elastic recoil of the lung, than in asthma.

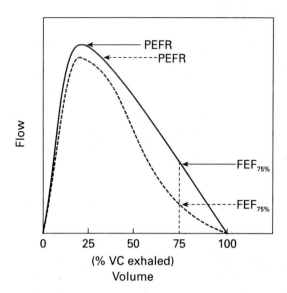

Figure 5. Maximum expiratory flow-volume (MEFV) curves in normal child (solid line) and child with small airways obstruction (dotted line) which is reflected by reduced $FEF_{75\%}$ but will not be apparent from PEFR unless there is secondary obstruction in the large airways.

The MEFV curve enables analysis of the effort-independent part of the FVC manoeuvre. This may have greater application to adult respiratory diseases than childhood asthma. However, it is an excellent method of assessing the reproducibility of FVC manoeuvres and whether a particular expiration is maximal (judged by the peak expiratory flow rate).

Peak expiratory flow rate

The peak expiratory flow rate (PEFR) is most accurately read off the MEFV curve. It is more usually estimated, however, using a portable dedicated flow meter such as the original Wright peak flow meter. It occurs very early in expiration and therefore does not require a prolonged expiratory manoeuvre making it easier for young children. It is also cheap to do. It has three determinants: the expiratory muscle strength; the expiratory effort; and the diameter of upper and large airways.

Summary of different parameters of an FVC manoeuvre

Each parameter reflects flow occurring at different times in the manoeuvre when lung volumes and the determinants of flow will differ. PEFR is the flow at high lung volume near to TLC and affected by large airway diameter. FEV_1 is the flow averaged over high and middle lung volumes. $FEF_{75\%}$ is the flow at low lung volume when the EPP has moved up the small airways and the flow is independent of effort. $FEF_{25-75\%}$ is the flow averaged over middle lung volume.

Measurement of static lung volumes

All the lung volumes (Figure 1) can be measured directly on a spirometer apart from residual volume which cannot be exhaled. The child needs to breathe quietly until a consistent baseline is achieved (at functional residual capacity) to indicate tidal breathing. A slow maximal expiration is then performed followed by a maximal inspiration or vice versa. Vital capacity measured this way should be equal to FVC but the latter may be slightly less as expiration is more likely to be incomplete.

RV, and therefore FRC and TLC, can only be measured by direct spirometry. In practice FRC is usually measured from which RV and TLC can be calculated. FRC is determined by a gas dilution technique or body plethysmography.

In the closed-circuit gas dilution technique a spirometer containing gas of known volume and helium concentration is connected to the child's lungs and allowed to equilibrate during tidal breathing. The FRC can then be calculated from the fall in helium concentration.

A body plethysmograph is an airtight box in which the subject sits breathing on a mouthpiece connected to the outside. The mouthpiece is occluded and the subject pants against it. Thoracic gas is then in an enclosed system with no air flow. Pressure changes measured at the mouth during panting therefore reflect those occurring on the whole system. According to Boyle's law the product of pressure and volume within the closed system should remain constant, or $P \times V = [P + \Delta P] \times [V + \Delta V]$. The change in volume in the system during panting will be the same as that observed in the plethysmograph. This is derived from the small change in pressure as this is another enclosed system. The thoracic gas volume can therefore be calculated. If the mouthpiece were occluded at end-expiration then this volume will be the FRC.

When there is airways obstruction such as in asthma, FRC measured by gas dilution may be underestimated because the helium will equilibrate less well in obstructed areas particularly where air is trapped. Plethysmography remains the 'gold standard' but even this can occasionally overestimate FRC if the subject develops acute bronchospasm because of the panting.

Tests for bronchial hyperresponsiveness

These tests look at the susceptibility to bronchoconstriction in response to provocation. Bronchoconstriction is usually gauged by a change in a parameter of forced expiratory flow. The provocation may be specific such as with an allergen but is more commonly nonspecific. Nonspecific bronchial hyperresponsiveness can be assessed with pharmacological agents such as histamine or methacholine, or by physical stimuli like exercise, cold air, hyperventilation or hypotonic nebulized fluids. Bronchoprovocation tests in children have largely been used as research tools but may have clinical value (Irwin and Pratter, 1990).

Pharmacological tests

Various methods of testing have been described but the principles are similar. Doubling concentrations of histamine or methacholine are inhaled starting with a very low dose and FEV_1 is measured after each dose. The agent may be inhaled by tidal breathing for a fixed period from a nebulizer, using a dosimeter or via a hand-activated nebulizer. The percentage fall in FEV_1 is plotted against the logarithm of the dose (when inhalation is inter-mittent) or the concentration (when inhaling continuously) of the challeng-ing agent. The dose or concentration required to produce a 20% fall from baseline FEV_1 is obtained by interpolation and used to express the degree of hyperresponsiveness. This is the provocative dose (PD_{20}) or provocative concentration (PC_{20}).

The method described by Cockcroft et al (1977) has been widely used but there are quicker methods (Yan et al, 1983) which appear to compare well (Britton et al, 1986).

Exercise tests

Exercise-induced symptoms are a common feature of childhood asthma. Exercise is more physiological than pharmacological challenging. Hyper-responsiveness to histamine or methocholine is common to asthma and many other chronic lung diseases in childhood and exercise-responsiveness may help to distinguish the two (Godfrey et al, 1991).

Exercise testing is not easily standardized and requires expensive equip-ment. A typical challenge may require the child to run at 5 km/hour on a treadmill inclined at $10°$ to raise the pulse to 160–180 beats/minute. FEV_1 is measured before and 3, 5, 10, 15 and 20 minutes after the onset of exer-cise. The result is expressed as the maximum percent fall in FEV_1 from baseline.

Performing lung function tests in children

Technique

Most of the tests which have been described above are dependent on the child's ability to perform maximal inspiration and expiration on demand. Few children under the age of 6 years will manage a reliable FVC manoeuvre although younger children may perform peak expiratory flow which does not require exhaling to residual volume (Milner and Ingram, 1970). In adults during an FVC test, expiration should be maintained for a minimum of 6 seconds (Gardner et al, 1987). However, 3 seconds may be acceptable in young children. Vociferous exhortation to keep blowing is frequently necessary.

Most children prefer to stand for an FVC manoeuvre. The spirometer must be brought down to a suitable height so that the neck is not extended as this can affect maximum expiratory flows (Melissinos and Mead, 1977). A child may not allow the application of a nose-clip and gently pinching the nose with one's fingers during the procedure can be useful. They should be able to see a real-time display of the manoeuvre as a source of encouragement and to allow an assessment of the adequacy of the effort (Becklake et al, 1991).

The best from a series of at least three acceptable measurements is conventionally taken as the definitive reading (Gardner et al, 1987). It should be noted, however, that when asked to give six consecutive peak expiratory flow measurements less than half of a group of asthmatic children recorded the highest reading in the first three blows (Greenough et al, 1990). No more than eight manoeuvres should be set as an upper limit (Kanner et al, 1983).

Preschool children and infants

Lung function testing in preschool children and infants who cannot even manage the peak expiratory flow manoeuvre generally requires the facilities and expertise of a specialized paediatric respiratory laboratory. Most of the tests do not yet have a place in the routine management of childhood asthma making detailed consideration beyond the scope of this chapter.

Some young children can be coached to perform tidal breathing on a spirometer and then a partial forced expiration. Even if the expiration does not begin at total lung capacity or end at residual volume, flow can be measured at a low lung volume such as end-tidal expiration, i.e. FRC, when it is independent of effort. Similar partial expiratory flow–volume curves can be generated in a baby by squeezing the chest with an inflatable jacket (Taussig et al, 1982). For lung volume measurements by gas dilution a mask would be substituted for a mouthpiece and a smaller volume spirometer and breathing circuit would be required but the principles are the same (Greenough et al, 1987).

Changes in oxygenation can be easily measured in infants and may reflect altered lung mechanics if this results in increased ventilation–perfusion mismatching. Transcutaneous oxygen tension has been proposed as an alternative to formal tests of lung function in methacholine challenge tests in very young children (Wilson et al, 1991). Oxygen saturation was not useful here although it was used in another study to monitor the response to a hypoxic provocation (Wagner et al, 1994). The assertion that children with reactive airways disease desaturate more readily to this challenge requires further evaluation.

Normal values

Ideally every lung function laboratory should select normal reference ranges from studies in a population typical of its patients. Once selected the range should be tested against 20–40 normal subjects before adoption. Discrepancies may not simply reflect an inappropriate range but may reveal errors from equipment or faulty technique.

Normal lung function is affected by a large number of factors. These include size, age, sex and race (Becklake et al, 1991) which should be taken into consideration. Height is the usual measure of size and is of particular importance in children. In children who are unable to stand upright armspan may be substituted (Hibbert et al, 1988). There are numerous studies showing racial differences in lung function (Schwartz et al, 1988; Greenough et al, 1991). Normal measurements in Caucasians tend to be higher than in other races and may be related to a higher trunk:leg ratio.

In clinical practice measurements in children are usually compared to published summary normal standards which pool data from many studies and do not distinguish sexes (Polgar and Promadhat, 1971). Standard curves giving a summary mean ± 2 standard deviations are given for all the common measures of lung volume and mechanics. Percentile growth curves for lung function parameters are now being published which have been calculated from data collected longitudinally in a consistent fashion (Dockery et al, 1983).

The common practice of expressing lung function results as a percent of the predicted mean value has been deplored in adults because a given percent value has different implications for different ages (Miller and Pinock, 1988). FEV_1 falls between the ages of 30–70 years but the variability is uniform. The percent predicted value which defines the fifth centile in men of height 1.7 metres at 30 years is 74% but at 70 years it is 63%! It is now recommended that normal ranges should be based on calculated fifth centiles rather than '80% of predicted' in adults (Becklake et al, 1991).

Fortunately in children, change in FEV_1 can be viewed in terms of increasing height and the scatter around the mean for FEV_1 decreases as the mean decreases (Dockery et al, 1983). Thus 80% predicted will define a similar centile at different heights and its use to distinguish the norm is probably justified (Quanjer, 1988). There would, however, be no more reason to express abnormal lung function in this way, than abnormal height or weight if centile charts were readily available.

ROLE OF LUNG FUNCTION TESTING

Lung function testing in childhood asthma provides an objective measure of different aspects of airways obstruction. These include the presence, degree and reversibility of airflow obstruction and the secondary effects such as air trapping and the propensity of the child towards its manifestation. The main applications are in diagnosis, determining severity and monitoring progress.

Diagnosis

It must be stressed that the diagnosis of asthma, particularly in childhood, is largely based on history. Any lung function tests which a child can manage are used to provide corroboration. Many asthmatic children will be too young to perform the standard tests. Furthermore, sophisticated testing with expensive equipment will only be appropriate for a small minority.

The American Thoracic Society (ATS) once defined asthma as 'a disease characterized by an increased responsiveness of the trachea and bronchi to various stimuli and manifested by widespread narrowing of the airways that changes in severity either spontaneously or as a result of therapy.' Individual lung function tests measure different aspects of this definition and no single test can therefore be diagnostic. Newer definitions recognize the presence of airways inflammation but whether any lung function testing can provide an indirect measure of inflammation is not certain.

Baseline spirometry and lung volumes, the acute response on spirometry to a bronchodilator and more long-term response to anti-asthma therapy, the monitoring of spontaneous airway lability in the course of a day, and bronchoprovocation tests each shed a different light in the diagnosis of the complex condition labelled asthma. Each will be considered in turn.

Baseline spirometry and lung volumes

If a child suspected of having asthma is capable of an FVC manoeuvre, spirometry is recommended in the initial assessment (Sheffer et al, 1992). FEV_1 is the most easily measured and reproducible parameter. A value well below the lower limit of normal for height suggests the presence of airways obstruction supporting a diagnosis of asthma.

Often, however, the interpretation will be less clearcut. Normal FEV_1 has a Gaussian distribution. Thus a value, for example on the 25th centile, may be normal for one child but indicate obstruction in another. There is no way of distinguishing from a one-off measurement. This again illustrates why expressing normality simply in terms of being greater than 80% predicted FEV_1 may be as unsatisfactory as applying this principle to the child's weight or height. Longitudinal testing comparing a child's own measurements over time is liable to be more informative than one comparison with the normal range.

Air flow obstruction in asthma is by definition variable and a child will frequently be in a remission phase at presentation in the clinic. Either way the baseline measurement is important in the diagnosis of asthma by demonstrating current airflow obstruction or enabling its demonstration by a future comparison.

A reduced FVC on spirometry in asthma can be interpreted as an indication of air trapping since it results from an increased FRC which may only be partially offset by an increased total lung capacity. At times, however, it may be useful to look for air trapping directly by measuring FRC and RV. A baseline demonstration of air trapping supports the diagnosis of asthma and provides another parameter by which the response to treatment may be monitored objectively in addition to spirometry. Some asthmatic children show persistent evidence of hyperinflation even during an asymptomatic phase (Pool et al, 1988). Occult pulmonary abnormalities not detected by forced breathing manoeuvres have been well documented (Cooper et al, 1977).

Reversibility of airways obstruction

Changes in airways narrowing as a result of therapy is a feature of asthma. Demonstrating an improvement in forced expiratory flow following inhalation of a bronchodilator is therefore diagnostically useful. The bronchodilator response can be assessed using peak flow rate, but FEV_1 is preferable as being a more reliable measure. Baseline FEV_1 is performed and repeated 5–15 minutes after inhalation of a bronchodilator, at or slightly over the usual therapeutic dose. The ATS recommendation for a significant response to bronchodilator in adults is a 12% or greater increase from baseline FEV_1 (Becklake et al, 1991). An increase of 8% or less was thought to be within the measurement variability. A recent International Consensus Report, however, recommended a greater than 15% increase as the guideline (Sheffer et al, 1992).

Unfortunately bronchodilator responsiveness is a very insensitive test for asthma. Children in an asymptomatic phase of episodic asthma or with relatively mild airways obstruction may be too close to maximal broncho-dilatation to give a significant response. At the other end of the spectrum, children with perennial asthma and persistent hyperinflation, but normal airway resistance, showed little reversibility to a bronchodilator (Kraemer et al, 1983).

In these children airways oedema and secretions may be of greater importance than any bronchoconstriction. Improvement in lung dynamics and volumes, and restoration of a bronchodilator response after a therapeutic trial of oral prednisolone, 1–2 mg/kg/day for 1 week, strongly supports the diagnosis of asthma. An alternative approach would be to look for improve-ment after treatment with an inhaled corticosteroid for 4–6 weeks.

Monitoring bronchial lability

Normal bronchomotor tone shows a diurnal circadian rhythmn so that expiratory flows are usually lowest in the early morning and highest in the afternoon. Increased bronchial lability refers to an exaggeration of these differences and is characteristic of asthma.

It is measured by monitoring the PEFR at least twice a day (morning and evening) for 1–2 weeks. Various ways of describing lability have been used. The percent lability can be calculated for each day by expressing the difference (or maximum difference if the PEFR is recorded more than twice daily) in PEFR divided by the mean PEFR as a percentage (Enright et al, 1994). Other denominators have been used; some use the mean PEFR over the whole period of monitoring (Hetzel and Clark, 1980) and the highest PEFR is recommended by others (Sheffer et al, 1992).

Defining normal lability in the face of diverse methods of calculation is not easy. Hetzel and Clark's (1980) suggestion of using > 20% (averaged over the monitoring period) as a useful screening test for asthma in adults is often quoted. However Johnston et al (1984) found the mean percent lability in a group of wheezy children (daily lability calculated according to our first definition above and averaged over the period of monitoring) was

17% (range 4–48%). They concluded that measuring lability would be too insensitive to have any diagnostic value for asthma in children.

More recently, an upper limit of normal (95th centile) percent lability for normal children aged 6–16 years has been quoted to be 31% (Quackenboss et al, 1991). In the same study excessive lability, defined as being over the 95th centile for more than 5% of the test days, was specific for asthma in children but had a sensitivity of only 60%. In other words 40% of asthmatic children would not have been picked up by the test.

Although cited here as an adjunct to the diagnosis of asthma it shares the problems of monitoring PEFR at home in general which are discussed in a later section.

Bronchoprovocation tests

In theory, if spirometry and lung volumes were normal, there was no bronchodilator response and no bronchial lability could be demonstrated, one might consider the remaining characteristic in the definition of asthma, i.e. 'increased responsiveness of the trachea and bronchi to various stimuli'. In clinical practice this approach is rarely productive.

Bronchial hyperresponsiveness is not specific for asthma as it has been well documented in many other respiratory disorders such as cystic fibrosis (Price et al, 1979), bronchopulmonary dysplasia (Smyth et al, 1981), post-bronchiolitis (Gurwitz et al, 1981) and even after upper respiratory infection (Empey et al, 1976). It has been suggested that bronchoprovocation may be better at 'ruling out' asthma than 'ruling it in' (Irwin and Pratter, 1990). Does a negative test 'rule out' asthma in the child with chronic respiratory symptoms, most usually cough in the clinical situation, when spirometry is normal? In one study 11% of a sub-group of children with chronic cough and negative methacholine challenge subsequently developed clinical asthma (Galvez et al, 1987).

Studies which compare bronchial responsiveness in subjects selected to be clearly asthmatic or clearly normal are bound to exaggerate the apparent discriminatory value of the test (Britton and Tattersfield, 1986). Its clinical value must therefore be judged in the clinical situation. It does not separate reliably asthmatic from nonasthmatic children in the general community (Salome et al, 1987; Pattemore et al, 1990). One of the difficulties may be its changeable nature. Thus bronchial hyperresponsiveness may only be guaranteed in asthma when measured during, or temporally close to, a symptomatic period (Cockcroft and Hargreave, 1990). However, in a longitudinal study where methacholine challenges were performed in asthmatic children and adults every 2–3 weeks over a year or more, exacerbations could occur in the absence of hyperresponsiveness (Josephs et al, 1989).

Bronchoprovocation tests have an important role in defining groups of children in asthma research. In clinical practice they may well have a role in the diagnosis of occupational asthma in adults (Irwin and Pratter, 1990). In children, their usefulness must be judged by their contribution when it may be difficult to make a diagnosis of asthma. On the present evidence this is not usually great.

Assessing severity

A child with moderate asthma could have a severe attack. Severity may therefore be considered in two ways: the severity of an individual attack and the severity of the disease generally. Lung function tests may be used to measure both.

The severity of an acute attack depends on the degree and extent of airways obstruction and therefore also on FEV_1 to which it is directly related (Enright et al, 1994). Again the importance of establishing a child's individual 'best lung function' against which the level during an exacerbation might be compared is emphasized. A particular value predicted for height may be normal for one child but represent considerable obstruction in another. The degree of air trapping as determined by measurement of residual volume also provides information on the severity of the deficit.

Severity of the disease is usually gauged by the amount of treatment required and the disruption to ordinary living. To an extent this will also vary with the degree of persistent airways obstruction. Attempts have been made to relate severity in adults to percent predicted FEV_1, TLC and VC but are not well standardized (Becklake et al, 1991). Furthermore, if the asthma is episodic rather than persistent, occasional lung function measurements in the clinic will not always reflect asthma severity between visits. A period of home monitoring (see below) might be more informative.

Bronchial hyperresponsiveness may be related to the degree of airway inflammation. PD_{20} (PC_{20}) has been proposed as another parameter by which asthma severity may be judged (Woolcock and Jenkins, 1990). In adults (Juniper et al, 1981) and children (Avital et al, 1991) the degree of hyperresponsiveness is higher in those judged to have more severe disease according to their drug requirements. However, there was considerable overlap between groups of different severity. It is also unclear whether bronchial hyperresponsiveness could be the cause or the manifestation of asthma severity.

Cockcroft and Hargreave (1990) assert that airway responsiveness should not be used to judge asthma severity but pose the possibility of its use as an index of airways inflammation and guide for anti-inflammatory treatment.

Monitoring

The diagnostic value of monitoring lung function (i.e. measuring the same parameter over a period of time) has been discussed. Monitoring has a greater role in assessing the response to treatment and dictating therapy. There are three main settings where this may be required: in the out-patient clinic or GP surgery; in the Accident and Emergency department and hospital ward; and at home. The facility and reliability of measurements in each setting will vary and will be discussed in turn.

Out-patient clinic/GP surgery

A recent international consensus statement (Sheffer et al, 1992) recommends spirometry for initial assessment of suspected asthma and subsequent monitoring in selected patients. PEFR measurement was considered the minimum objective parameter for monitoring and making therapeutic decisions. This may be appropriate for the GP surgery or relatively mild asthmatics. Readings made on mini flow meters must be interpreted with caution as they are often inaccurate. They tend to read low flows quite well, over-read flows between 200 and 400 l/minute (the usual paediatric range) and under-read higher flows (Miller et al, 1992). Readings vary between different brands of flow meter and to make comparisons over time it would be desirable to use the same meter such as the child's own meter (Sly et al, 1994). In asthmatic children who warrant hospital out-patient follow-up and can manage an FVC manoeuvre it would be preferable to use FEV_1 for monitoring.

PEFR is not a substitute for FEV_1 because they measure different things. The peak flow occurs within the FEV_1 so it is not surprising that the two are highly correlated. However, the fallacy of equating correlation with equivalence has been eloquently demonstrated by Bland and Altman (1986). A significant discrepancy in terms of the percent predicted value has been found to exist between estimations of PEFR and FEV_1 in stable asthmatic children suggesting that the former may underestimate the degree of airway patency in this situation (Meltzer et al, 1989).

It can be argued that using a post-bronchodilator FEV_1 to compare lung function between clinic visits, rather than the baseline FEV_1, would control for variables such as the time elapsed since the last medication, recent allergen exposure, time of day, etc. which may affect the latter measurement (Enright et al, 1994).

Accident and emergency department/hospital ward

During an acute asthma attack, lung function estimations can help to guide treatment. Airways obstruction would not be subtle and would not be hidden within a PEFR measurement. Being the most portable, easiest and cheapest of the standard tests, PEFR monitoring is the method of choice in the emergency situation when a rough indication of gross change is all that is required. It enables objective assessment of the response to nebulized bronchodilator, whether hospital admission is indicated and how aggressive subsequent therapy should be. It also provides objective documentation of improvement on the ward which would influence the timing of discharge.

Published guidelines for the management of acute severe asthma in children urge no other investigation before instigating treatment (British Thoracic Society et al, 1993). They recommend measuring PEFR before and 15–30 minutes after the first nebulised β-agonist to help decide the course of subsequent treatment. They suggest monitoring PEFR before and after nebulizers at least four times daily throughout the hospital stay. The significance of different measurements is given in terms of percent predicted for height or percent of a known best recording. Obviously the latter would be preferable as discussed previously.

Home monitoring

Asthma is a disease of variable airways obstruction. Normal lung function at two clinic visits may be associated with considerable derangement between the visits. This illustrates again that lung function tests are an adjunct to clinical history and examination in the management of children with asthma. However parents' perception of airways obstruction in their children may not be reliable (Sly et al, 1985). Measuring lung function at home should provide more objective evidence of airways obstruction from day to day. Currently the only practical means of home monitoring is by PEFR using mini flow meters. The child's PEFR is measured usually twice daily, in the morning and evening before any medication, and the readings are recorded in a diary with space to enter use of bronchodilators and symptoms.

There are a few specific instances when keeping a PEFR diary for short (1–2 weeks) periods may be useful. Its diagnostic use in revealing bronchial lability and its use in assessing asthma severity, particularly when the history is unclear, have been mentioned earlier. It can also be used for close observation of the effect of a change in treatment.

More extended monitoring may provide evidence of airways obstruction not apparent at clinic visits. The promotion of continual PEFR monitoring coincides with the emergence of self-management plans for asthma. These involve a patient or the parents adjusting treatment depending on PEFR measurements according to previously set guidelines. For example colour-coded PEFR zones might be established to indicate different action: green for 80–100% of best PEFR indicating routine treatment; yellow for 50–80% of best PEFR indicating specified increases in treatment; and red for below 50% of best PEFR indicating urgent treatment and medical assistance (Sheffer et al, 1992).

Although widely advocated for all patients on maintenance treatment, these plans have only really been evaluated in adults and many of the studies showing benefit are uncontrolled (Beasley et al, 1989). Indeed the case against wholesale monitoring is strengthening. PEFR monitoring with self-management guidelines conferred little benefit in a recent randomized-controlled trial in over 500 adult patients in north-east Scotland (Drummond et al, 1994).

There is less information on continual home PEFR monitoring in children. However, twice daily recordings in a relatively asymptomatic child may be a greater burden to the child than the disease. Clinicians who care for asthmatic children will be familiar with a small number of parents who become obsessed with their child's PEFR to the exclusion of common sense. However, most parents find PEFR monitoring of greater use in assessing asthma severity during symptoms than detecting asthma when asymptomatic (Lloyd and Ali, 1992). Perhaps continual monitoring should be reserved for children and particularly adolescents with severe brittle asthma where early warning of deterioration may be important. The Scottish study may have demonstrated greater benefit from PEFR monitoring if only severe asthmatic patients had been included. Intermittent monitoring may be more appropriate for the majority of asthmatic children on regular treatment. This does not preclude a self-management plan based on knowledge of the best PEFR when well, and the level which should prompt action.

Attention must be given to the reliability of PEFR diary entries in studies on home monitoring. An ingenius study using electronic recording devices in asthmatic adults demonstrated that a significant proportion of entries in diary cards were invented or retrospective (Chowienczyk et al, 1994). There is little reason to believe that a busy parent or young adolescent would be more concientious. Of even greater concern is the findings of a study where recording was reliable, being made in a boarding school by the the investigators rather than parents. PEFR monitoring failed to detect over half of clinically important reductions in lung function demonstrable on spirometry over 3 months (Sly et al, 1994). A considerable number of false-positive reductions were also seen with all of the four brands of mini flow meters used. While the routine use of continual PEFR monitoring is unlikely to benefit the majority of asthmatic children, even in those with severe asthma, a number of questions remain over its efficacy.

SUMMARY

Asthma is mainly a disorder of expiration. Airways obstruction causes dynamic airways compression earlier in expiration leading to air trapping and hyperinflation. Tests of forced expiration indicate the presence and degree of airways obstruction by reduced flow. They are the easiest and most useful tests of lung function. However, few children under 6 years will manage an FVC manoeuvre. Asthma in children is largely a clinical diagnosis but lung function tests can provide useful corroborative information. Assessing bronchial responsiveness has diagnostic value in research but rarely in the clinical setting. It may provide an index of airways inflammation which would have therapeutic implications. FEV_1 is the best parameter for routine monitoring in the hospital clinic. PEFR is not a substitute for FEV_1. It is useful in the emergency situation but the reliability of home PEFR monitoring needs further evaluation.

REFERENCES

Avital A, Noviski N, Bar-Yishay E et al (1991) Nonspecific bronchial reactivity in asthmatic children depends on severity but not on age. *American Review of Respiratory Disease* **144:** 36–38.

Beasley R, Cushley M & Holgate ST (1989) A self management plan for the treatment of adult asthma. *Thorax* **44:** 200–204.

Becklake M, Crapo RO, Buist S et al (1991) Lung function testing: selection of reference values and interpretative strategies. Official statement of the American Thoracic Society. *American Review of Respiratory Disease* **144:** 1202–1218.

Blackie SP, Al-Majed S, Staples CA et al (1990) Changes in total lung capacity during acute spontaneous asthma. *American Review of Respiratory Disease* **142:** 79–83.

Bland JM & Altman DG (1986) Statistical methods for assessing agreement between two methods of clinical measurement. *The Lancet* **i:** 307–310.

British Thoracic Society, British Paediatric Association, Research Unit of the Royal College of Physicians of London et al (1993) Guidelines on the management of asthma. *Thorax* **48**: S1–S24.

Britton J & Tattersfield (1986) Does measurement of bronchial hyperreactivity help in the clinical diagnosis of asthma? *European Journal of Respiratory Disease* **68**: 233–238.

Britton J, Mortagy A & Tattersfield A (1986) Histamine challenge testing: Comparison of three methods. *Thorax* **41**: 128–132.

Chowienczyk PJ, Parkin DH, Lawson CP & Cochrane GM (1994) Do asthmatic patients correctly record home spirometry measurements? *British Medical Journal* **309**: 1618.

Cockcroft DW & Hargreave FE (1990) Airway hyperresponsiveness. Relevance of random population data to clinical usefulness. *American Journal of Respiratory Disease* **142**: 497–500.

Cockcroft DW, Killian DN, Mellon JJ et al (1977) Bronchial reactivity to inhaled histamine: A method and clinical survey. *Clinical Allergy* **7**: 235–243.

Cogswell JJ, Hull D, Milner AD et al (1975) Lung function in childhood I. The forced expiratory volumes in healthy children using a spirometer and reverse plethysmograph. *British Journal of Diseases of the Chest* **69**: 40–50.

Cooper DM, Crutz E & Levison H (1977) Occult pulmonary abnormalities in asymptomatic children. *Chest* **71**: 361.

Dockery DW, Berkey CS, Ware JH et al (1983) Distribution of forced vital capacity and forced expiratory volume in one second in children 6 to 11 years of age. *American Review of Respiratory Disease* **128**: 405–412.

Drummond N, Abdalla M, Beattie JAG et al (1994) Effectiveness of routine self monitoring of peak flow in patients with asthma. Grampian Asthma Study of Integrated Care. *British Medical Journal* **308**: 564–567.

Empey DW, Laitinen LA, Jacobs L et al (1976) Mechanisms of bronchial hyperactivity in normal subjects after upper respiratory infection. *American Review of Respiratory Disease* **113**: 131.

Enright PL, Lebowitz MD & Cockcroft DW (1994) Physiologic measures: pulmonary function tests. Asthma outcome. *American Journal of Respiratory and Critical Care Medicine* **149**: S9–S18.

Galvez RA, McLaughlin FJ & Levison H (1987) The role of the methacholine challenge in children with chronic cough. *Journal of Allergy and Clinical Immunology* **79**: 331–335.

Gardner RM, Hankinson JL, Clausen JL et al (1987) Standardization of spirometry—1987 update. Official statement of the American Thoracic Society. *American Review of Respiratory Disease* **136**: 1285–1298.

Godfrey S, Springer C, Noviski N et al (1991) Exercise but not methacholine differentiates asthma from chronic lung disease in children. *Thorax* **46**: 488–492.

Greenough A, Everett L & Price JF (1990) Are we recording peak flows properly in young children? *European Respiratory Journal* **3**: 1193–1196.

Greenough A, Loftus BG, Pool J & Price JF (1987) Abnormalities of lung mechanics in young asthmatic children. *Thorax* **42**: 500–505.

Greenough A, Hird MF, Everett L & Price JF (1991) Importance of using lung function regression equations appropriate for ethnic origin. *Paediatric Pulmonology* **11**: 207–211

Gurwitz D, Mindorff C & Levison H (1981) Increased incidence of bronchial reactivity in children with history of bronchiolitis. *Journal of Pediatrics* **98**: 551.

Hetzel MR & Clark TJH (1980) Comparison of normal and asthmatic circadian rhythms in peak expiratory flow rate *Thorax* **35**: 732–738.

Hibbert ME, Lanigan A, Raven J & Phelan PD (1988) Relation of armspan to height and the prediction of lung function. *Thorax* **43**: 657–659.

Hutchison AA, Erben A, McLennan LA et al (1981) Intrasubject variability of pulmonary function testing in healthy children. *Thorax* **36**: 370–377.

Irwin RS & Pratter MR (1990) The clinical value of pharmacologic bronchoprovocation challenge. *Medical Clinics of North America* **74**: 767–778.

Johnston I, Anderson HR & Patel S (1984) Variability of peak flow in wheezy children. *Thorax* **39**: 583–587.

Josephs LK, Gregg I, Mulee MA & Holgate ST (1989) Nonspecific bronchial reactivity and its relationship to the clinical expression of asthma. *American Review of Respiratory Disease* **140**: 350–357.

Juniper EF, Frith PA & Hargreave FE (1981) Airways responsiveness to histamine and methacholine: relationship to minimum treatment to control symptoms of asthma. *Thorax* **36**: 575–579.

Kanner RE, Schenker MB, Munoz A & Speizer FE (1983) Spirometry in children: methodology for obtaining optimal results for clinical and epidemiological studies. *American Review of Respiratory Disease* **127**: 720–724.

Kraemer R, Meister B, Schaad UB & Rossi E (1983) Reversibility of lung function abnormalities in children with perennial asthma. *The Journal of Paediatrics* **102**: 347–350.

Krowka MJ, Enright PL, Rodarte JR & Hyatt RE (1987) Effect of effort on measurement of forced expiratory volume in one second. *American Review of Respiratory Disease* **136**: 829–833.

Lloyd BW & Ali MH (1992) How useful do parents find home peak flow monitoring for children with asthma. *Thorax* **305**: 1128–1129.

Melissinos CG & Mead J (1977) Maximum expiratory flow changes induced by longitudinal tension on trachea in normal subjects. *Journal of Applied Physiology* **43**: 537–544.

Meltzer AA, Smolensky MH, D'Alonzo GE et al (1989) An assessment of peak expiratory flow as a surrogate measurement of FEV_1 in stable asthmatic children. *Chest* **96**: 329–333.

Miller MR & Pincock AC (1988) Predicted values: how should we use them? *Thorax* **43**: 265–267.

Miller MR, Dickinson SA & Hitchings DJ (1992) The accuracy of portable peak flow meters. *Thorax* **47**: 904–909.

Milner AD & Ingram D (1970) Peak expiratory flow rates in children under 5 years of age. *Archives of Disease in Childhood* **45**: 780–782.

Pattemore PK, Asher MI, Harrison AC et al (1990) The interrelationship among bronchial hyperresponsiveness, the diagnosis of asthma, and asthma symptoms. *American Review of Respiratory Disease* **142**: 549–554.

Polgar G & Promadhat V (1971) *Pulmonary Function Testing in Children: Techniques and Standards*. Philadelphia: WB Saunders.

Pool JB, Greenough A & Price JF (1988) Abnormalities of functional residual capacity in symptomatic and asymptomatic young asthmatics. *Acta Paediatrica Scandinavica* **77**: 419–423.

Price JF, Weller PH, Harper SA & Matthew DJ (1979) Response to bronchial provocation and exercise in children with cystic fibrosis. *Clinical Allergy* **9**: 563–570.

Quackenboss JJ, Lebowitz MD & Krzyzanowski M (1991) The normal range of diurnal changes in peak expiratory flow rates: relationship to symptoms and respiratory disease. *American Review of Respiratory Disease* **143**: 323–330.

Quanjer PH (1988) Predicted values: how should we use them? [letter]. *Thorax* **43**: 663–664.

Salome CM, Peat JK, Britton WJ & Woolcock AJ (1987) Bronchial hyperresponsiveness in two populations of Australian schoolchildren. I. Relation to respiratory symptoms and diagnosed asthma. *Clinical Allergy* **17**: 271–281.

Schwartz JD, Katz SA, Fegley RW & Tockman MS (1988) Sex and race differences in the development of lung function. *American Review of Respiratory Disease* **138**: 1415–1421.

Sheffer AL (chairman), Bousquet J, Busse WW et al (1992) International consensus report on diagnosis and treatment of asthma. *European Respiratory Journal* **5**: 601–641.

Sly PD, Landau LI & Weymouth R (1985) Home recording of peak expiratory flow rates and perception of asthma. *American Journal of Disease in Childhood* **139**: 479–482.

Sly PD, Cahill P, Willet K & Burton (1994) Accuracy of mini peak flow meters in indicating changes in lung function in children with asthma. *British Medical Journal* **308**: 572–574.

Smyth JA, Tabachnik E, Duncan WJ et al (1981) Pulmonary function and bronchial hyperreactivity in long-term survivors of bronchopulmonary dysplasia. *Pediatrics* **68**: 336.

Taussig LM, Landau LI, Godfrey S & Arad I (1982) Determinants of forced expiratory flow in newborn infants. *Journal of Applied Physiology* **53**: 1220–1227.

Wagner CL, Brooks JG, Richter SE et al (1994) The '88% saturation test': A simple lung function test for young children. *Pediatrics* **93**: 63–67.

West JB (1987) *Pulmonary pathophysiology—the essentials*, 3rd ed. Baltimore: Williams and Wilkins.

Wilson NM, Phagoo SB & Silverman M (1991) Use of oxygen tension, arterial oxygen saturation and respiratory resistance to assess the response to inhaled methacholine in asthmatic children and normal adults. *Thorax* **46**: 433–437.

Woolcock AJ & Jenkins CR (1990) Assessment of bronchial responsiveness as a guide to prognosis and therapy in asthma. *Medical Clinics of North America* **74**: 753–765.

Yan K, Salome C & Woolcock AJ (1983) A rapid method for measurement of bronchial hyperresponsiveness. *Thorax* **38**: 760–765.

7

Management of acute asthma in children

ALAN F. ISLES
CHRISTOPHER J. L. NEWTH

This chapter presents recommendations for the management of acute asthma in children and reviews information in three areas: (1) drug delivery to the respiratory tract; (2) the pharmacology of asthma medications; and (3) the assessment and treatment of acute asthma.

DRUG DELIVERY TO THE RESPIRATORY TRACT

Inhaled therapy

Administration of medication by inhalation allows direct targeting of the medication to the site of action. Lower doses can be used and the risk of significant systemic side effects is reduced. A full discussion of all aspects of aerosol therapy is beyond the scope of this review. Only those aspects relevant to the treatment of acute asthma in children will be discussed. Other aspects of aerosol therapy have been reviewed in detail by Newman (1991), Dolovich and Newhouse (1993) and Bisgaard (1994).

Jet nebulizers

Jet nebulizers are an efficient way of delivering drugs to the lungs but pumps are expensive, cumbersome and require a power supply. Furthermore, the performance of nebulizing systems varies widely resulting in differing output of particles within the respirable range and in the percentage of the drug available for delivery to the lung. The effective dose delivered by the nebulizer is determined by a number of factors, including the efficiency of the compressor, the type of nebulizer and the fill volume (Dolovich and Newhouse, 1993). The output and efficiency of both compressors and nebulizers deteriorates with continued use (Bisgaard, 1994). Hardy et al (1993) reported that the effective dose delivered by different nebulizers can vary by as much as 10-fold. A fill volume of 3–5 ml usually results in maximal response (Dolovich and Newhouse, 1993). About two-thirds of the aerosol is lost, as inspiration occupies only one-third of the respiratory cycle. Bisgaard (1994) reported that 68% of the dose remains behind in the nebulizer and only 11–14% of the dose is nominally available for inhalation. In addition, if the face mask is loosely-fitting, the delivered dose is further reduced by as much as 50% and Bisgaard estimated that with the way most nebulizer treatments are given to children only about 5% of the nominal dose is inhaled. O'Callaghan (1993) suggested that a struggling un-cooperative child may receive very little of the prescribed medication. Silverman (1990) has also argued that, in a quietly breathing young infant, drug delivery by jet nebulizer is negligible. Other reports (Collis et al, 1990; Bisgaard, 1994) suggest that after 6 months of age the quantity of aerosol inspired from a jet nebulizer is largely independent of age due to entrainment which occurs when inspiratory flow exceeds jet-nebulizer output.

Metered dose inhalers (MDIs) with spacers have begun to displace jet nebulizers in the home management of acute asthma. MDIs and small-volume spacer (Aerochamber®, Baby-Spacer® or Baby-haler®) are an effective alternative to jet nebulizers in infants. Jet nebulizers are never required in the daily management of most older children with stable asthma who are capable of using alternative delivery devices. Jet nebulizers continue to play an important role in the management of acute asthma in the hospital setting.

Metered dose inhalers

The usefulness of MDIs in children is limited by a range of problems including incorrect co-ordination of inhalation and MDI actuation, cessation of inhalation when the cold aerosol particles reach the palate and too rapid inhalation (Pedersen, 1994). Optimal aerosol delivery is achieved when the dose is delivered at the beginning of a slow deep inhalation followed by a 10s breath-hold (Vidgren, 1994). At faster inhalation rates, the clinical efficacy of bronchodilator drugs can be reduced by 50% (Newman and Pavia, 1985). More than 50% of children use MDIs incorrectly thus reducing the benefit from prescribed medication (Pedersen et al, 1986). Conventional MDIs cannot therefore be recommended for use in children when alternative devices are available (O'Callaghan, 1993; Pedersen, 1994). For young children, an MDI should always be combined with a large-volume spacer. After appropriate tuition, children over 7 years of age may be able to use an MDI for relief of minor symptoms but most will benefit from the addition of a spacer for relief of acute symptoms. Use of a breath-actuated MDI (Autohaler®) eliminates the difficulies with co-ordination of acuation and inhalation but the other MDI-related problems remain and the Autohaler® should be reserved for children greater than 6–7 years of age (Pedersen, 1994).

Metered dose inhaler plus spacer

Delivery of medication by an MDI and spacer has advantages over delivery by jet nebulizer. The devices are portable, cheap and easier to use and maintain. Spacers overcome the problem of co-ordination of aerosol actuation and dose delivery and reduce oro-pharyngeal impaction (Vidgren,

1994). Because treatment is simpler compliance may also improve. Most children over 2–3 years of age can be trained to use a large-volume spacer (Pedersen, 1994). As with an MDI, a slow deep inhalation from a spacer is preferable (Bisgaard, 1994). In younger children, tidal breathing on the spacer is satisfactory. O'Callaghan (1993) has suggested that at low tidal volumes the high aerosol concentration in small-volume spacer devices enhances the amount of drug available for inhalation, while at higher tidal volumes the amount of drug available may be greater from large-volume spacers. Some younger children may be unable to manage an MDI and spacer in the presence of acute asthma and treatment with a jet nebulizer may be necessary (Pedersen, 1994).

Most currently available spacer devices were designed for use in older children and must be adapted for use in infants and younger children. Bisgaard (1994) described an age-dependency of dose delivery through large and small-volume spacers. Although theoretical models have predicted an increased lung deposition in infants due to smaller airway calibre and greater ventilation/kg body weight (Phalen et al, 1988; Hofmann et al, 1989), measurement of the nominal dose available from these devices in infants suggests otherwise (Bisgaard, 1994). The use of a standard large-volume spacer with an attached face-mask for use in infants typically results in a reduction in the dose available for delivery to the airway. Most standard spacers have inadequate valving arrangements for infants. The valve either does not open if the inspiratory pressure is too low or, alternatively, does not close, allowing expiration back into the chamber, thus expelling aerosol. During inspiration, air may also be entrained around a loose fitting mask or through the expiratory side-port in the mouth piece further reducing the inspired dose (Bisgaard, 1994). The volume of the spacer is also critical in determining the effective dose. Small-volume spacers are more easily emptied but also result in greater impaction of aerosol particles and increased sedimentation thus reducing the available dose. The optimal size of the spacer for infants is thus a balance between these two issues. Bisgaard (1994) has recently evaluated a two-way, low resistance small-volume spacer and compared it with a standard large-volume spacer with face mask. Drug delivery from the large-volume spacer was reduced from 42% in older children to 20% in infants whilst the small-volume valved spacer delivered 38% of the dose regardless of age. The clinical efficacy of a similar small-volume valved spacer for administering salbutamol to wheezy infants has been reported by Kraemer et al (1991) and by Clarke et al (1993).

Dry powder inhalers

Dry powder inhalers (DPIs) have become more popular with the introduction of multi-dose devices and because of the need to remove CFC propellants from MDIs. The advantages of the DPI are that it is breath-actuated overcoming the co-ordination problems involved with standard MDIs, especially in children. New generation dry powder devices such as the Turbuhaler® have proven efficacy in adults and older children.

However, the inspiratory flow required for optimal use is 30–60 l/minute (Bisgaard, 1994). In contrast to MDIs, a fast inhalation is required with the DPI for optimal delivery (Pedersen et al, 1990). Several studies have demonstrated that a considerable number of children below 7 years of age are unable to achieve the minimal inspiratory flow required and indiscriminate use of these devices in younger children cannot be recommended (Bisgaard, 1994). Some younger children may use the device successfully when they are well but not in the presence of acute asthma.

Pulmonary deposition varies markedly according to the delivery device used (Derom et al, 1994). After Agertoft and Pedersen (1993) demonstrated that the dose of budesonide required to maintain good asthma control when administered by an MDI and spacer could be reduced by half when given by Turbuhaler® without loss of symptom control and attributed this effect to greater pulmonary deposition from the Turbuhaler®.

Other routes of administration

Oral route

Oral bronchodilators are virtually never indicated in the treatment of acute symptoms in children. The previously limited role of oral bronchodilators in infants and young children has been largely eliminated by the use of an MDI with small-volume spacers and face masks in this age group. However, oral corticosteroids have become a central element of most protocols for the treatment of acute asthma.

Parenteral route

A more aggressive approach to the use of inhaled β_2- adrenergic agonists and the declining role of aminophylline in the treatment of acute asthma have resulted in a much reduced need for parenteral therapy in the majority of children admitted with acute asthma. Parenteral corticosteroids may be required if gastro-intestinal intolerance prevents use of oral corticosteroids. Parenteral administration of β_2-adrenergic agonists may be necessary in the intensive care management of critically ill patients.

PHARMACOLOGY OF ASTHMA MEDICATIONS

β-adrenergic agonists

The β_2-adrenergic agonists are the most effective bronchodilators currently available. The structure and function of the β_2-adrenergic receptor have been defined (Fraser et al, 1993), and the molecular mechanisms underlying the bronchodilator activity of β_2-adrenergic agonists have recently been elucidated (Barnes and Lee, 1992). The β_2-adrenergic agonists cause bronchodilatation by activation of a large conductance calcium-activated potassium channel, known as the maxi-K channel (Small et al, 1993). Blocking the maxi-K channel with charybdotoxin blocks the bronchodilator activity of β_2-agonists in both animal and human airways (Barnes and Lee, 1992). Activation of the β_2-receptor results in increased intracellular cyclic-AMP concentrations which, in turn, activate the maxi-K channel by phosphorylation (Small et al, 1993). There is also evidence that the β_2-receptor is directly coupled to the maxi-K channel via a stimulatory G protein without the involvement of the second messenger cyclic-AMP (Small et al, 1993). Potassium channel opening results in cellular hyperpolarization and inhibition of calcium influx (Small et al, 1993).

The mechanism of action of long-acting β_2-adrenergic agonists such as salmeterol and formoterol is similar to the short-acting β_2-adrenergic agonists. Johnson (1992) originally proposed that their long duration of action was explained by their binding to an exo-site allowing the active saligenin end of the molecule to interact repeatedly with the β-receptor. More recently, Anderson et al (1994) proposed that the extended duration of action of this class is determined principally by their physicochemical interaction with membrane lipid bi-layers.

The β_2-adrenergic agonists have a range of other effects, some of which are relevant to their use in acute asthma. Following reports from New Zealand of an apparent increase risk of death in patients using β_2-agonists, there have been continuing concerns about the potential for adverse effects from β_2-adrenergic agonists (Beasley et al, 1991). This issue and the potential mechanisms have been reviewed in detail by Morley et al (1990), Warner (1994), Sterk (1994) and McFadden (1994b). Mullen et al (1993) performed a meta-analysis of the published case-controlled studies and reported that the relationship between β-agonist use and death from asthma was weak and of small magnitude. The adverse cardiac effects of therapeutic doses of β_2-adrenergic agonists appear to be relatively minor but it is possible that the hypercapnia, hypoxia, and hypokalaemia encountered in acute asthma may magnify these effects (Warner, 1994). Continued administration of high doses of β_2-adrenergic agonists produces hypokalaemia through the stimulation of the adenosine triphosphate system causing potassium to move into cells. DuPlooy et al (1994) have also shown that acute administration of salbutamol can also cause hyperkalaemia. Chronic use of β_2-adrenergic agonists can also increase bronchial reactivity (Warner, 1994). Other potential interactions between β_2-adrenergic agonists and corticosteroids are discussed in the section on corticosteroids.

The possible role of airway smooth muscle β_2-adrenoceptor dysfunction in the pathogenesis of asthma remains uncertain (Bai et al, 1992). In severe or fatal asthma, a decreased relaxant response to β_2-adrenoceptor agonists has been reported with an apparent correlation between the degree of β_2-adrenoceptor hypofunction and the severity of the asthma (Cerrina et al, 1986). Bai et al (1992) evaluated the β_2-adrenergic affinity and density in airway smooth muscle of subjects with fatal asthma. They found no evidence of a decrease in receptor density but did observe a reduced functioning of the β_2-adrenoceptors and speculated that this was due to an uncoupling of the receptors from other elements of the relaxant system induced by products of the inflammatory process.

From a practical point of view, for the treatment of acute asthma, β_2-adrenergic agonists should be given by inhalation. Occasionally, in critically-ill patients, parenteral administration is required (see section on intensive care management). β_2-adrenergic agonists can be given by inhalation using pressurized MDI (preferably with attached spacer), DPI, or jet nebulizer. The relative advantages and disadvantages of each have been reviewed earlier in the section on drug delivery.

Dry powder inhalers have significant limitations in the treatment of acute asthma in children, especially in the younger age-groups (Pederson et al, 1990). High inspiratory flow rates are required to deliver effectively the powder from these devices. Generation of these flow rates may be difficult during an acute exacerbation, especially in younger children. Alternative delivery devices are recommended for children younger than about 6 years of age.

Metered dose inhalers combined with a large-volume spacer are displacing nebulizers for the home treatment of acute asthma symptoms. A number of studies (Idris et al, 1993; Kerem et al, 1993) have shown this combination to be as effective as a jet nebulizer for acute asthma. The dose administered is dependent on weight. The dose administered by Kerem et al (1993) was six puffs of salbutamol for children < 25 kg in weight, eight puffs for those 25–35 kg and 10 puffs for those > 35 kg. Spacers have also been used successfully to deliver β_2-agonist to infants (Conner et al, 1989; Bisgaard, 1993).

Jet nebulizers remain the mainstay for treatment of acute asthma in the hospital setting. Dosage recommendations vary widely. Robertson et al (1985) demonstrated the superior efficacy of frequent small doses of salbutamol (0.15 mg/kg given every 20 minutes) compared to the same total dose given hourly. Schuh et al (1989, 1990) then demonstrated the safety and efficacy of higher doses (0.3 mg/kg) given in the same manner. Oberklaid et al (1993) demonstrated that a fixed dose (2.5 mg) of salbutamol was as effective as a dose calculated on body weight. As clinical experience with more aggressive use of β_2-agonists has grown, administration of continuous nebulized β_2-adrenergic agonist is now widely recommended for the treatment of severe acute asthma in children (Warner, 1992). Katz et al (1993) and Singh and Kumar (1993) have reported on the safety and efficacy of continuous nebulized β_2-adrenergic agonist in infants and children. Continuous nebulized treatment has reduced the need for intravenous treatment even in hypercapnic acute asthma (Salmeron et al, 1994).

Theophylline

Theophylline has been used in the treatment of asthma for over 50 years and, because of its low cost, remains one of the most widely prescribed anti-asthma medications (Barnes and Pauwels, 1994). In recent years, with more effective use of inhaled bronchodilator therapy, the role of theophylline, especially in the management of acute asthma, has declined. Some have even suggested that it is obsolete.

Mechanism of action

The precise mechanism of action at a cellular level remains unclear (Barnes and Pauwels, 1994) and it is possible that several different mechanisms are operative:

(i)   phosphodiesterase inhibition;
(ii)   adenosine receptor blockade;
(iii) increase in circulating adrenaline;
(iv)   mediator antagonism;
(v)   inhibition of calcium ion flux.

Current knowledge regarding each of these potential mechanisms of action has been reviewed by Barnes and Pauwels (1994). Theophylline is conventionally regarded as exerting its effects by phosphodiesterase (PDE) inhibition. However, PDE activity is only modestly reduced (5–20%) by therapeutic concentrations of theophylline (Bergstrand, 1980). Elevation of cyclic-AMP by β-agonists may result in increased PDE activity (Barnes and Pauwels, 1994). This may mean that theophylline has a greater than expected inhibitory effect on PDE in asthmatics taking β_2-adrenergic agonists regularly than in normals. A lack of any bronchodilator effect of theophylline in normal subjects has been previously reported (Estenne et al, 1980). Furthermore, inhibition of PDE could lead to synergistic interaction with β_2-adrenergic agonists (Barnes and Pauwels, 1994).

Theophylline is a potent adenosine receptor antagonist at therapeutic concentrations and this, most probably, accounts for many of the side effects of theophylline, such as central nervous system stimulation, cardiac arrhythmias, gastric hypersecretion, gastro-oesophageal reflux and diuresis (Barnes and Pauwels, 1994). Therapeutic concentrations of theophylline inhibit the bronchoconstrictor effect of adenosine (Mann and Holgate, 1985) but the relevance of this observation to the anti-asthma effects of theophylline remain unclear (Barnes and Pauwels, 1994).

Intravenous aminophylline has an acute bronchodilator effect in asthmatic patients and a satisfactory risk benefit ratio is achieved with concentrations in the range of 10–20 mg/l (Mitenko and Ogilvie, 1973). However, the bronchodilator effects of theophylline in chronic asthma are small when compared to β_2-adrenergic agonists, leading to speculation that theophylline has other anti-asthma effects which are also important (Pauwels and Persson, 1991). Theophylline has anti-inflammatory effects that are therapeutically relevant (Barnes and Pauwels, 1994). There is also evidence that theophylline opens large conductance calcium-activated potassium channels (maxi-K channels) in the airway smooth muscle cell membrane via an increase in cyclic-AMP (Jones et al, 1990). This is similar to the putative mechanism of action of β-agonists (Barnes and Pauwels, 1994). There is now evidence that β-adrenoreceptors in airway smooth muscle of patients with fatal asthma become 'un-coupled' (Bai et al, 1992). In airways obtained at postmortem, the relaxant effect to β-agonists is reduced, whereas the bronchodilator response to theophylline is maintained (Goldie et al, 1986). These data suggest that theophylline may be useful in acute asthma, especially if the response to β₂-adrenergic agonists is poor (Barnes and Pauwels, 1994).

An effect of theophylline which remains controversial is its action on respiratory muscles. Aminophylline increases diaphragmatic contractility and reverses diaphragmatic fatigue (Aubier et al, 1981). This effect has often been used to support the use of aminophylline in acute severe asthma with impending respiratory failure. However, the significance of the effect of aminophylline on the diaphragm has been questioned by Maxham (1988) and by Jenne (1994).

Use of aminophylline in acute severe asthma

More aggressive use of nebulized bronchodilator therapy in recent years has led to a re-examination of the role of aminophylline in acute asthma. In patients with acute asthma, intravenous aminophylline is less effective as a bronchodilator than β-agonists (Bowler et al, 1987). A meta-analysis of suitably designed studies comparing β-agonists with and without intravenous aminophylline showed no additional benefit from adding intravenous aminophylline (Wrenn et al, 1991). Zainudin et al (1994) similarly showed no added benefit from the combined treatment.

Carter et al (1993) treated 21 children aged 5–18 years with acute asthma and showed that theophylline, at therapeutic concentrations, did not give additional benefit to children hospitalized with acute asthma who were treated with frequent doses of nebulized albuterol (salbutamol) and with intravenous methylprednisolone. Di Guilio et al (1993) drew similar conclusions from an acute study in 29 children. Weinberger (1993) in a commentary on these two studies noted that both studies excluded those who were progressing to respiratory failure despite vigorous use of inhaled β₂-adrenergic agonists and systemically administered steroids and speculated that this may have biased the outcome against theophylline.

Current opinion suggests that intravenous aminophylline should not be added routinely in the treatment of acute asthma. It should be reserved for the few patients with acute severe asthma who fail to show a satisfactory response to frequent doses of nebulized bronchodilator and oral or parenteral steroids (Jenne, 1993; Weinberger, 1993; Barnes and Pauwels, 1994).

Therapeutic range

The usually accepted therapeutic range of 10–20 mg/l was based on measurements of the acute bronchodilator response to aminophylline administered intravenously in acute asthma (Mitenko and Ogilvie, 1973). Adverse effects can occur at concentrations within this range and Barnes and Pauwels (1994) argue that side effects can be reduced by aiming for a plasma concentration of 5–15 mg/l rather than the previously recommended range of 10–20 mg/l.

Interactions

A range of factors decrease theophylline clearance necessitating a dose reduction. Hendeles et al (1992) reviewed the safety and efficacy of theophylline in children with asthma and provided a full review of the interactions. Important interactions in the treatment of patients with acute asthma include a reduction in theophylline clearance by viral infections and interactions with erythromycin, cimetidine, ciprofloxacin and carbamazepine.

Use of intravenous aminophylline

Current guidelines recommend an initial loading dose should be administered to achieve a serum concentration within the therapeutic range. The usual loading dose of aminophylline is 6 mg/kg but this needs to be reduced if the patient has previously been taking theophylline. In this situation, it is preferable to measure the serum theophylline concentration before giving further aminophylline. If a serum concentration cannot be readily obtained, the loading dose should not exceed 3 mg/kg. As an approximation, each 1 mg/kg of aminophylline will give a 2 mg/l, increase in serum concentration.

Following the loading dose, a maintenance dose infusion of 1.5 mg/kg/hour in 1–9-year-old children and 1.2 mg/kg/hour in the 10–16 year age group should be used. Lower doses are required in the first year of life (0.5 mg/kg/hour). Serum theophylline concentrations should be monitored at regular intervals, e.g. at 1, 12 and 24 hours after commencing the infusion to ensure maximum therapeutic benefit and to minimize the risk of toxicity. Treatment should be discontinued if the serum concentration exceeds 20 mg/l (Murphy and Kelly, 1991).

Anticholinergic drugs

The role of the cholinergic nervous system in normal and asthmatic airways has been reviewed by Barnes (1993) and Widdicombe (1993). Cholinergic nerve fibres travel down the vagus nerve and synapse in para-sympathetic ganglia which are located within the airway wall. From these ganglia, short post-ganglionic fibres travel to airway smooth muscle and mucus glands. The cholinergic nervous system controls resting bronchomotor tone. Cholinergic innervation is greatest in large airways and diminishes peripherally and, as expected, cholinergic bronchoconstriction predominantly involves large central airways (Barnes, 1993). The relative diminution of cholinergic control in small airways may have important clinical implications since anticholinergic drugs are likely to be less useful than β_2-adrenergic agonists when bronchoconstriction involves small airways (Barnes, 1993).

Cholinergic effects on the airways are mediated via muscarinic receptors on target cells in the airways. At least five sub-types of muscarinic receptor have been described (Widdicombe, 1993). Cholinergic bronchoconstriction can be triggered by a variety of stimuli including the mediators released in asthmatic inflammation (Barnes, 1993).

The pharmacology of anticholinergic drugs has been reviewed by Gross (1988) and by Bauer and Banholzer (1993). Current anticholinergic agents are not selective in action and block all types of muscarinic receptors. Anticholinergic drugs block the muscarinic action of acetylcholine at receptors on post-synaptic membranes (Gross, 1988). Ipratropium bromide and oxtropium are derivates of atropine with poor lipid solubility which, when taken by inhalation, have local anticholinergic effects in the airway and cause few systemic effects (Gross, 1988).

Cumulative dose-response testing of ipratropium bromide in children using doses ranging from 75 to 250 μg demonstrated a plateau in the dose-response curve within this dose range and 250 μg has been recommended as the optimal dose for children (Davis et al, 1984).

As expected with a blocking drug, tolerance or tachyphylaxis does not occur (Barnes, 1991). The safety and side effects of anticholinergic bronchodilators have been reviewed by Gross (1993). The role of ipratropium bromide in the treatment of acute asthma in children has been reviewed by Henry (1990) and Reisman et al (1993). Studies by Beck et al (1985) and Reisman et al (1988) demonstrated that the combination of ipratropium bromide and salbutamol was more effective than salbutamol alone in children with acute asthma treated in the Emergency Room. By contrast, others have found no benefit from the combined therapy (Storr and Lenney, 1986). Reisman et al (1993) observed that since completion of their studies with combination therapy, the use of β-adrenergic agonists in acute asthma has altered with larger and more frequent doses being used and they question whether ipratropium is of added benefit when maximal doses of β-adrenergic agonist are given. When used in combination with a β-adrenergic agonist, Reisman et al (1993) recommend 125 μg for children under 4 years of age and 250 μg in older children administered hourly if necessary until the patient has improved.

The role of ipratropium in the treatment of infants has been examined by Stokes et al (1983) and by Naspitz and Sole (1992).

Corticosteroids

Glucocorticosteroids are the most potent anti-inflammatory drugs used in the treatment of acute asthma exacerbations. There is now an improved understanding of their mechanism of action, especially at a cellular level (Miesfeld, 1990; Barnes and Adcock, 1993; Taylor and Shaw, 1993).

Glucocorticoids (GC) exert their effects on cells by binding to a cyto-plasmic glucocorticoid receptor (GCR). There appears to be a single class of GCR and no evidence of differing receptor sub-types with differing affinities in different cells (Brattsand, 1992). The GCR has several distinct structural and functional domains (Barnes and Adcock, 1993). The cortico-steroid binding site is at the C-terminal end of the molecule. Adjacent to this is the tau-2 domain which is important to nuclear localization of the activated receptor. The DNA-binding region in the centre of the molecule is folded into two long 'zinc fingers' which serve to aid linkage between the GCR and the DNA. The N-terminal end is involved with transcriptional activity once DNA binding occurs.

The inactive GCR is bound to a protein complex which includes two heat-shock proteins bound at the C-terminal end (Barnes and Adcock, 1993). It is thought that the role of heat-shock protein is to facilitate the proper folding of the GCR into a conformation optimal for binding with GC and also prevent the GCR from localizing into the nucleus (Munch et al, 1990). Once GC binds to the GCR, the heat-shock protein dissociates and the activated GCR forms a dimer and moves rapidly into the nucleus where it binds to specific glucocorticoid-responsive elements (GREs) on DNA and is then able to exert wide ranging anti-inflammatory effects by stimulating or inhibiting the production of proteins in target genes. The effects of GC have been reviewed by Barnes and Adcock (1993) and include the following.

(a)   Inhibition of the formation of a range of cytokines including interleukins 1 and 3–8, and tumour necrosis factor -alpha.
(b)   Inhibition of the formation of certain cytokine receptors, e.g. the interleukin-2 receptor.
(c)   They act directly on other transcription factors to counteract the cellular effects of cytokines.
(d)   Increased synthesis of lipocortin-1 which has an inhibitory effect on phospholipase A2 thereby inhibiting the production of lipid mediators such as leukotrienes, prostaglandins and platelet activating factor.
(e)   Enhancement of the metabolism of mediators such as bradykinin by inducing the activity of the degrading enzyme.
(f)   A direct inhibitory effect on the expression of adhesion molecules on endothelial cells which recruit other inflammatory cells.
(g)   Decreased microvascular permeability (Williams and Yarwood, 1990).
(h)   Decreased mucus secretion in asthmatic airways (Lundgren et al, 1990).

There are also important interactions between CS and the β-adrenergic receptor. The gene for the β-adrenergic receptor has at least three GREs in its promoter sequence and CS increase synthesis of the receptor. There are also suggestions of a negative interaction between the two (Barnes and Adcock, 1993). They report evidence that a high concentration of β-agonist may interfere with the binding of the activated GCR to the GRE on DNA and this is one possible mechanism by which β-agonists may have harmful effects in asthma (Barnes and Adcock, 1993).

Corticosteroid resistance in asthma is an area of increasing interest and concern. Recent reviews of this subject include those of Tattersfield and Barnes (1992), Kamada et al (1992) and Cypar and Busse (1993). Kamada et al (1994) recently reported on the coexistence of GCR and pharmacokinetic abnormalities in children with steroid unresponsive asthma.

The pharmacokinetics of systemically administered corticosteroids have been evaluated (Hill et al, 1990). However, there is a poor understanding of the dose-response relationship of systemic corticosteroids in acute asthma. Measuring the plasma concentration of CS is largely irrelevant when CS act on a range of second-messenger systems and this is reflected in the time-lag between drug administration and clinical response. Littenberg and Gluck (1986) and Storr et al (1987) suggested that the time-lag between administration of CS and clinical effect could be as short as 3–4 hours but the more conventional view is that the time-lag is of the order of 6–12 hours (McFadden, 1994b). The literature on the dose-response relationship has been reviewed by Strauss et al (1990), Barnes (1992) and McFadden (1994a). Against this background, the reader should be aware that recommendations regarding optimal doses are empiric. When parenteral CS are used, there is no convincing evidence that high doses are more effective than lower doses (McFadden, 1994a; Bowler et al, 1992) or that methylprednisolone is more effective than hydrocortisone (Barnes, 1992). Storr et al (1987) and Connett et al (1993) reported that a single dose of prednisone was effective treatment for many children with acute asthma and reduced admission rates and improved recovery. However, another study by Ho et al (1994) could not confirm this observation. For oral corticosteroids in children, Phelan (1992) has recommended prednisone 1 mg/kg daily (to a maximum dose of 50 mg) for 3–5 days. For most acute episodes, extended tapering courses are not necessary. A longer course may be required when the acute episode occurs on a background of severe unstable asthma.

The role of inhaled steroids in the treatment of acute exacerbations remains unclear. Through many of the consensus statement guidelines it has become a recommended practice to double the dose of inhaled steroids during acute exacerbations. Although some studies have reported that inhaled steroids can prevent viral-induced exacerbations of asthma in children (Connett and Lenney, 1993), the evidence to support this as routine practice in children with acute asthma exacerbations is lacking. A recent study in adults by Greening et al (1994) raises further questions about the efficacy of an increased dose of inhaled steroids in controlling an exacerbation. Oral and inhaled steroids may have a complementary role. Jenkins and Woolcock (1988) demonstrated that inhaled but not oral steroids decrease airway reactivity. Dolan et al (1987) reported that even short courses of corticosteroids (less than 7 days) may place children at risk of adrenal insufficiency if more than four courses are given per year.

ASSESSMENT AND TREATMENT OF ACUTE ASTHMA IN CHILDREN

Acute exacerbations of asthma are responsible for more hospital admissions and missed school-days than any other chronic disease of childhood (Murphy and Kelly, 1991). The recent increase in asthma prevalence (Robertson et al, 1991; Peat et al, 1994) has been accompanied by an increase in hospital admissions for acute asthma (Hyndman et al, 1994). Some studies have suggested that the apparent increase in admissions is due to diagnostic transfer (Carmen and Landau, 1990) while other studies have suggested a real increase in both hospital admissions and in asthma severity (Kun et al, 1993).

Importantly, acute asthma can on occasions be fatal. The mortality rate from asthma in children is 0.6–0.9 per 100 000 population per year (Robertson et al, 1992). Studies of deaths from asthma in both adults and children have shown that the majority occur because of chronic undertreatment and sub-optimal management of an acute asthma attack due to a combination of factors including poor patient understanding, delay in seeking medical attention, and poor medical management of the acute attack (Sears, 1987). However, Robertson et al (1992) found that 33% of deaths in young people occurred in those judged to have mild asthma with no obvious additional risk factors. Most deaths from acute asthma occur prior to the person reaching a clinic or hospital (Murphy and Kelly, 1991).

Batty et al (1994) surveyed adults admitted to hospital with acute asthma and showed, using a morbidity scoring index, that most patients were at risk from asthma-associated morbidity because of poor levels of knowledge about their disease and its treatment. Canny et al (1989) examined the records of 1864 children who had 3358 presentations to the Emergency Room of a large tertiary paediatric hospital. They found that the mean duration of symptoms prior to presentation was 41 hours, 26% of the children required admission and 0.5% required admission to Intensive Care. History and clinical examination indicated that preceding respiratory infection was the cause of acute asthma in 75% of visits, supporting the contention that respiratory infection is the most common trigger for acute episodes of asthma in childhood (Conway and Littlewood, 1985). The study by Canny et al (1989) also emphasized that even in a major tertiary paediatric facility, appropriate recording of physical signs and measurements of lung function in children presenting to the Emergency Room with acute asthma was sub-optimal. They also observed that bronchodilators were given in sub-optimal doses and that corticosteroids were underutilized in the treatment of acute exacerbations.

Pathophysiology of acute asthma

The pathophysiological events in acute asthma are the result of airway narrowing secondary to bronchial smooth muscle constriction, inflammation and oedema of the bronchial mucosa, mucus secretion and epithelial shedding (Bone and Burch, 1991; McFadden 1994a). This airway narrowing is widespread but unevenly distributed resulting in an imbalance between ventilation and perfusion. In acute asthma, airway narrowing causes closure of small airways at higher than normal lung volumes. This, in turn, results in hyperinflation of the lung in order to increase elastic recoil pressure on the airways to aid expiration. Tonic contraction of inspiratory and accessory muscles during expiration contribute to hyperinflation during acute asthma (Bone and Burch, 1991). This dynamic hyperinflation of the lung to assist expiration places the inspiratory muscles at a significant disadvantage.

The combination of airway obstruction and hyperinflation results in a marked increase in the work of breathing (Permutt, 1973). In addition, hyperinflation impairs the efficiency of the diaphragm (Bone and Burch, 1991). As lung volume increases, the muscle fibres of the diaphragm shorten (reducing their force of contraction) and the radius of curvature of the diaphragm decreases, thereby decreasing its ability to exert pressure for a given force. Inspiratory airflow resistance is also increased as is the physiological dead-space, further increasing the work of breathing. These abnormalities in lung mechanics are manifested as a reduction in forced vital capacity (FVC) and forced expiratory volume (FEV_1) and a marked increase in residual volume and total lung capacity.

Uneven distribution of the airway narrowing causes ventilation–perfusion ($\dot{V}/\dot{Q}$) mismatching and resultant hypoxaemia. This $\dot{V}/\dot{Q}$ imbalance is the major mechanism impairing the efficiency of pulmonary gas exchange in acute asthma (Bone and Burch, 1991). $\dot{V}/\dot{Q}$ mismatching can be quantified noninvasively using an argon freon-22 re-breathing technique (Yiallouos and Milner, 1994). In a mild asthmatic attack, the primary gas exchange defect is hypoxaemia accompanied by hypocapnia, the latter reflecting the increased alveolar ventilation. As airflow obstruction increases, hypoxaemia increases and carbon dioxide levels initially normalize then increase. In general, carbon dioxide retention is not seen until the FEV_1 is about 15–20% of predicted normal (McFadden, 1994a).

The altered pulmonary mechanics and associated pressure swings cause decreased venous return during expiration and increased venous return during inspiration resulting in relative over-filling of the right ventricle (Bone and Burch, 1991). This causes a septal shift towards the left ventricle and impedes its filling. Systolic left ventricular ejection is decreased by the after-load created by the negative pleural pressure. The nett effect of this is a drop in systolic blood pressure during inspiration. This decrease in inspiratory blood pressure is known as pulsus paradoxus. There is general agreement that when pulsus paradoxus is present the magnitude of the pulsus paradoxus correlates with the severity of airflow obstruction. However, on occasions, severe airflow obstruction can be present without a significant increase in pulsus paradoxus.

Management of acute exacerbations

Exacerbations of asthma are acute or sub-acute episodes of progressively worsening shortness of breath, wheezing, chest tightness and cough, or some combination of these symptoms. Respiratory distress is also common. Exacerbations are characterized by decreases in expiratory flow which can be quantified by measurement of lung function (FEV_1 or peak expiratory flow). These objective measures, especially FEV_1, are more reliable indicators of the severity of an exacerbation than symptoms. The severity of an exacerbation may range from mild to life-threatening. Deterioration usually occurs over hours or days, but may occasionally occur precipitously over minutes. Morbidity and mortality are most often associated with under-assessment of the severity of the exacerbation, inadequate action at the onset of symptoms, and under-treatment of the exacerbation (International Consensus report on Diagnosis and Treatment of Asthma, 1992). A failure to make objective measurements has been recognized as a common problem in the assessment of acute asthma.

The goals of treatment of an acute exacerbation are: (a) to assess correctly the severity of the episode; and (b) to assign therapy appropriate for the degree of severity in order to provide relief of symptoms and to improve lung function as quickly as possible with minimal side effects.

Home-based treatment of the child with acute asthma

For those patients previously diagnosed with asthma, the first steps in treatment of an exacerbation will usually be taken at home as part of the individual's Asthma Management Plan. Early recognition of trigger factors and deterioration in asthma accompanied by a prompt intensification of treatment will frequently prevent or abort an acute exacerbation.

The essential elements of this approach are:

(i)   to educate all children with asthma, or their parents, to recognize early deterioration of their asthma;
(ii) for all children with asthma to have an Asthma Management Plan to guide prompt intensification of treatment; and
(iii) to promote prompt communication between patient and doctor and to have priority access to the local hospital Emergency Room.

The primary goal of home management of acute exacerbations is to avoid delays in instituting treatment. A secondary goal is for patients skilled in self-management to acquire a sense of control over their lives and their illness (Sheffer, 1991). It is equally important that the patient does not delay seeking medical help when the exacerbation is severe or if the response to treatment is not prompt and sustained. The home management strategy must be individualized and will depend on the skill and competence of the patient, or parents, and their access to emergency care.

Frequently, patients and parents recognize acute asthma as a sudden 'attack' without recognizing the more gradual increase in symptoms and decline in lung function which precedes the acute event (Stempel and Redding, 1992). The Asthma Management Plan should emphasize detection of the early warning signs of an acute exacerbation. Beer et al (1987) reported that prodromal symptoms were present for 6 hours or more in 71% of children who presented with acute asthma. In the other 29% of children, the acute exacerbation evolved within 6 hours. More importantly, they reported that the prodromal symptoms were the same on each occasion creating the opportunity for parents to react when they first recognize the prodromal symptoms rather than waiting for the onset of asthma symptoms.

Measurement of peak flow can be useful in home monitoring but peak flow meters can be inaccurate and not detect exacerbations (Sly et al, 1994).

Readings are effort-dependent and may be inaccurate, especially in young children and symptom-based Asthma Management Plans are generally preferred in children. A suggested protocol for the home management of acute exacerbations is shown in Figure 1.

If there is no improvement within 1 hour or if the conditions worsen, home treatment should not be continued. A need for increasingly frequent doses of bronchodilator and a decreasing response, indicate a need for urgent medical attention. Those who have previously had sudden severe attacks should proceed to hospital early after initiating treatment.

Hospital-based assessment and management of the child with acute asthma

Initial assessment

A brief history and physical examination are usually appropriate prior to initiating treatment. However, if the patient is acutely distressed, treatment with oxygen and inhaled β_2-adrenergic agonist should be given immediately.

Initial history. Important questions to ask include the following.

  (i) Duration of symptoms (with increasing duration of the attack, exhaustation and muscle fatigue may precipitate respiratory failure).
 (ii) Cause of present exacerbation of asthma. Ask about specific triggers such as infection, allergen exposure, aspirin, foods etc.
(iii) Severity of symptoms, including exercise limitation and sleep disturbance prior to presentation.
 (iv) All current medications, doses and amounts used including time of last dose/s.
  (v) Prior hospitalizations and emergency department visits for asthma, particularly within the past year.
 (vi) Prior episodes of severe life-threatening asthma especially intensive care admission and/or ventilation.
(vii) Any pre-existing cardiopulmonary disease.

An important function of this initial history is to identify patients at high-risk from their asthma. One or more of the following characteristics are usually present.

  (i) Current use of, or recent withdrawal, from oral corticosteroids.
 (ii) A history of admission to Intensive Care or a previous near-fatal attack.
(iii) Night time attacks, especially associated with severe chest tightness or 'choking'.
 (iv) Inadequate treatment or poor compliance with medical treatment programs, especially in teenagers or young adults.
  (v) Failure to perceive asthma symptoms, e.g. poor spirometry when patient denies symptoms.
 (vi) Denial of the diagnosis of asthma or other overt psychosocial problems.

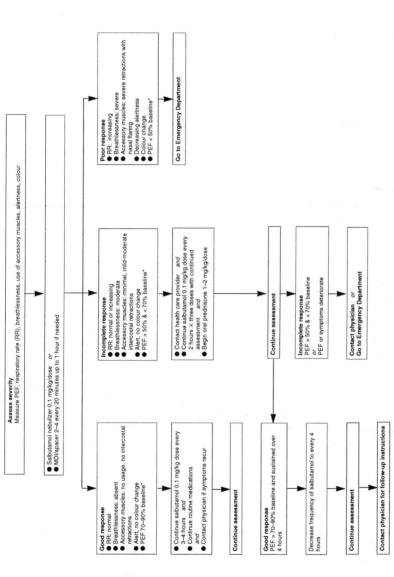

Figure 1. Acute exacerbations of asthma in children: home management. Reproduced from *Guidelines for Diagnosis and Management of Asthma* (1991, Bethesda: National Institutes of Health) with permission.

* PEF % baseline refers to the norm for the individual, established by the clinician. This may be % predicted based on standardized norms or % patient's personal best.

A more detailed history (see Appendix) and complete physical examination should be performed once therapy has been initiated and the patient's condition stabilized.

Rapid physical examination. A rapid cardio-pulmonary examination should be performed to evaluate the severity of the exacerbation and to identify major complications. The following should be specifically looked for:

(i) cyanosis;
(ii) tachycardia > 120/minute in older children and > 160/minute in young children;
(iii) inability to speak in sentences;
(iv) absence of wheezing may be a sign of severe airflow obstruction;
(v) use of accessory respiratory muscles;
(vi) physical evidence of a significant complication, e.g. subcutaneous emphysema, and a significant differential reduction of breath sounds, suggesting mucus plugging or pneumothorax;
(vii) pulsus paradoxus > 20 mmHg. However, the absence of pulsus paradoxus does not exclude a severe exacerbation.

Wheezing is the least sensitive indicator of airflow obstruction and of response to therapy.

Accessory muscle use correlates well with airway obstruction in children. It has been shown that the use of the sternocleidomastoid muscles correlates with a peak expiratory flow or FEV_1 of less than 50% of that predicted (Coomey and Levison, 1976)

When practical, objective measurements of airway function such as spirometry or peak flow should always be performed and be repeated after treatment to assess response. Admission to hospital is likely to be necessary if the post-bronchodilator peak expiratory flow (PEF) is < 60% of the child's previous best. It is not an appropriate time during an acute attack of asthma to teach a child how to use a peak flow meter. However, it may be worth attempting to obtain a reading since a normal value is reassuring but low readings may reflect poor technique rather than severe airflow obstruction (Henry et al, 1993). Measurement of PEF is effort-dependent and readings are unlikely to be reliable in sick, young children, and marginally useful even in children up to the age of 12–14 years when they are acutely unwell.

Pulse oximetry is now widely available in Emergency Departments and can be a useful adjunct to assessment, especially in the younger child. Geelhoed (1988) found the initial oximetry measurement to be a useful predictor of severity. If the oxygen saturation on arrival is 90% or less, admission is usually necessary and supplemental oxygen should always be administered. Many children with higher readings may also require admission (Henry et al, 1993). Pulse oximetry is not without problems, with many errors made by failure to ensure that the signal is adequate (Grace, 1994). The measured pulse rate should correlate with the pulse on the signal. Movement artefact, especially in young children, is a common cause for unreliable readings. When supplemental oxygen is used, normal oximetry readings can occur in the presence of respiratory failure (Henry et al, 1993).

Because of $\dot{V}/\dot{Q}$ abnormalities in infants, hypoxia will develop earlier than in older children or adults with a similar degree of obstruction and they can progress rapidly to respiratory failure. Pulse oximetry is recommended in infants presenting with an acute exacerbation (Boner et al, 1993). Isles and Newth (1993) have reviewed the management of wheezing in infants and provided specific protocols for management of acute episodes in this age group.

Measurement of arterial blood gases is not routinely necessary in the management of mild to moderate asthma exacerbations. Measurements are generally indicated in severe asthma where initial aggressive therapy has failed or the patient is critically ill on arrival. Treatment should not be delayed in order to perform these investigations.

Similarly, a chest X-ray is not routinely indicated in children presenting with acute asthma (Gershel et al, 1983; Henry et al, 1993). Obtaining a chest X-ray often involves moving the child to a different patient area where additional delays may occur and, unless appropriate monitoring is maintained, this can be hazardous. X-rays should be obtained selectively when there are focal physical signs which persist after treatment or clinical evidence of a major complication, such as pneumothorax or lung collapse (Henry et al, 1993). Treatment should not be delayed by performing unnecessary investigations.

The purpose of this initial rapid history and examination is to assess the severity of the episode and assign appropriate treatment. In general, children presenting to the Emergency Room with acute asthma can be divided into three categories: (i) those who can probably manage at home; (ii) those who require treatment in the Emergency Room and may subsequently require admission, and (iii) those who definitely require admission to hospital (*Asthma Management Handbook*, 1993) and these categories form a useful basis for treatment recommendations (see Table 1).

There are many acceptable protocols for the management of acute asthma and treatment practices vary somewhat between countries. Protocols based on a contemporary approach to treatment include those of Henry et al (1993), the International Consensus Report on Diagnosis and Management of Asthma (1992) and that of the British Thoracic Society (1993).

An approach to the Emergency Room management of acute asthma is shown in Figure 2. If discharge from the Emergency Room is considered the child should be observed for a minimum of 60 minutes after the last dose of medication. The decision to admit or discharge should be based on objective measures such as respiratory rate and spirometry or peak flow. Relief of wheezing is not a reliable indicator of response to treatment. The child should not be discharged unless the expectation is that they will not require bronchodilator given more often than every 3 hours (Henry et al, 1993). At discharge, the child or parent must be given instructions for continuing medication and advised to seek medical review in the next 24 h. A significant exacerbation requiring presentation to hospital also indicates a need to review and, if necessary, modify both the daily maintenance program and the Asthma Management Plan.

With mild to moderate exacerbations there are no absolute rules as to

Table 1. Initial assessment of severity of asthma in children.

	Probably manage at home	May need hospital admission	Admission required
Altered consciousness	No	No	Yes
Physical exhaustion	No	No	Yes
Ability to talk	Sentences	Phrases	Words
Pulsus paradoxus	Not palpable	May be palpable	Usually palpable
Central cyanosis	Absent	Absent	Present
Wheeze on auscultation	Present	Present	May be absent
Use of accessory muscles	Absent	Moderate	Marked
Sternal retraction (in young children)	Absent	Moderate	Marked
Peak flow after initial treatment % predicted or % personal best	> 70–80%	50–70%	< 50%
Oximetry on presentation prior to treatment (SaO_2)	> 93%	91–93%	90% or less

Reproduced from the *Asthma Management Handbook* (1993, Melbourne: National Asthma Campaign) with permission.

who should be admitted to hospital and this decision will be influenced by a range of factors, both medical and social. Factors which favour hospital admission include:

—inadequate response to therapy after 1–2 hours of treatment;
—persisting severe airflow limitation (PEF < 40% of predicted or personal best);
—past history of severe asthma requiring admission;
—presence of high risk factors (see previous list);
—prolonged symptoms before the current exacerbation and presentation;
—geographical isolation from emergency care;
—psychosocial factors.

Bollinger et al (1992) reviewed the relationship between various measures of asthma severity and outcome in severe acute asthma. They reviewed most of the previously published literature on scoring systems and use of specific indices which might predict who can be discharged from the Emergency Room and those who will almost certainly require admission. No single measure proved universally successful in predicting the need for admission. Some useful recommendations can be made however. In children, even if wheeze has been relieved, discharge from the Emergency Room is unwise if tachypnoea persists (Henry et al, 1993). Similarly, discharge with an FEV_1 or PEF of < 50% is likely to lead to early return. An approach to the in-patient management of children with acute asthma is shown in Figure 3.

The child's condition should be re-evaluated on admission to the ward. The importance of repeated objective measurements of pulse rate, respiratory rate and peak flow (in older children) in assessing the child's progress and response to medication cannot be over-emphasized.

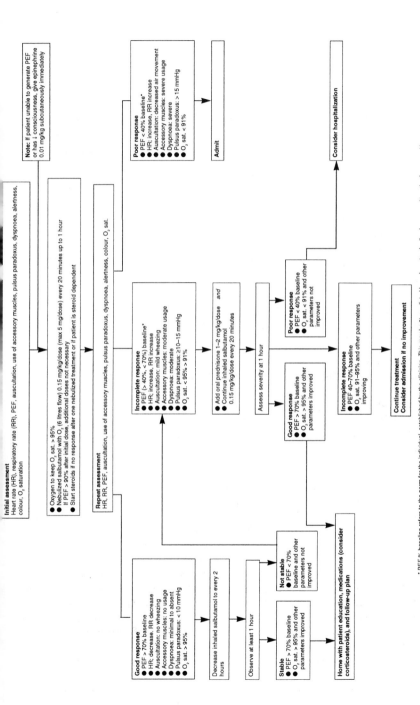

Figure 2. Acute exacerbations of asthma in children: Emergency Department management. Reproduced from *Guidelines for Diagnosis and Management of Asthma* (1991, Bethesda: National Institutes of Health) with permission.

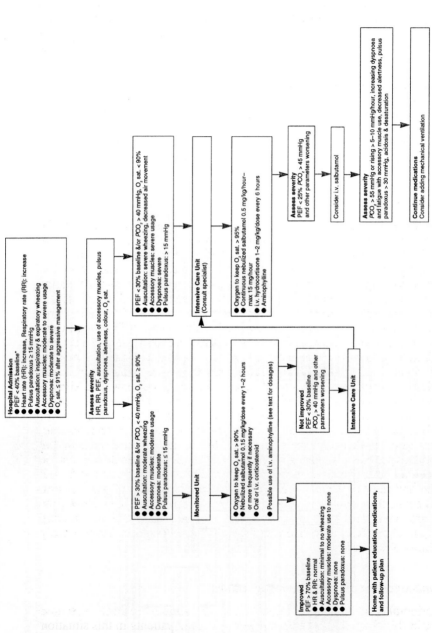

Hospital Admission
- PEF <40% baseline*
- Heart rate (HR): increase, Respiratory rate (RR): increase
- Pulsus paradoxus ≥ 15 mmHg
- Auscultation: inspiratory & expiratory wheezing
- Accessory muscles: moderate to severe usage
- Dyspnoea: moderate to severe
- O₂ sat. ≤ 91% after aggressive management

Assess severity
HR, RR, PEF, auscultation, use of accessory muscles, pulsus paradoxus, dyspnoea, alertness, colour, O₂ sat.

- PEF > 30% baseline &/or PCO₂ < 40 mmHg, O₂ sat. ≥ 90%
- Auscultation: moderate wheezing
- Accessory muscles: moderate usage
- Dyspnoea: moderate
- Pulsus paradoxus: ≤ 15 mmHg

- PEF < 30% baseline &/or PCO₂ > 40 mmHg, O₂ sat. < 90%
- Auscultation: severe wheezing, decreased air movement
- Accessory muscles: severe usage
- Dyspnoea: severe
- Pulsus paradoxus: > 15 mmHg

Monitored Unit

Intensive Care Unit
(Consult specialist)

- Oxygen to keep O₂ sat. > 90%
- Nebulized salbutamol 0.15 mg/kg/dose every 1–2 hours or more frequently if necessary
- Oral or i.v. corticosteroid
- Possible use of i.v. aminophylline (see text for dosages)

- Oxygen to keep O₂ sat. > 95%
- Continuous nebulized salbutamol 0.5 mg/kg/hour– max 15 mg/hour
- i.v. hydrocortisone 1–2 mg/kg/dose every 6 hours
- Aminophylline

Improved
PEF > 70% baseline
- HR & RR: normal
- Auscultation: minimal to no wheezing
- Accessory muscles: moderate use to none
- Dyspnoea: none
- Pulsus paradoxus: none

Not Improved
PEF < 30% baseline
PCO₂ > 40 mmHg and other parameters worsening

Assess severity
PEF < 30% baseline &/or PCO₂ > 45 mmHg and other parameters worsening

Intensive Care Unit

Home with patient education, medications, and follow-up plan

Consider i.v. salbutamol

Assess severity
PCO₂ > 55 mmHg or rising > 5–10 mmHg/hour, increasing dyspnoea and fatigue with accessory muscle use, decreased alertness, pulsus paradoxus > 30 mmHg, acidosis & desaturation

Continue medications
Consider adding mechanical ventilation

* PEF % baseline refers to the norm for the individual established by the clinician. This may be % predicted based on standardized norms or % patient's personal best.

Figure 3. Acute exacerbations of asthma in children: hospital management. Reproduced from *Guidelines for Diagnosis and Management of Asthma* (1991, Bethesda: National Institutes of Health) with permission.

Criteria for admission to the Intensive Care Unit

Criteria for admission are generally nonspecific and rely on care givers having a high index of suspicion for impending respiratory failure (understanding the limited physiological and anatomical reserves of sick infants and children with asthma) and a low threshold for aggressive therapeutic intervention. Some cautionary features include:

previous history of respiratory failure;
drug toxicity (e.g. sedating agents or theophylline);
other medical conditions likely to be aggravated by asthma drug therapy
    (e.g. supraventricular tachycardia);
exhaustion (e.g. altered level of consciousness, lethargy, diaphoresis);
an elevated and/or rising carbon dioxide tension despite implementation of
    adequate standard therapy;
air-leak syndromes;
cardiac or respiratory arrest.

Specific methods of evaluation are available that allow assessment of the severity of an attack and the likelihood of admission to the Intensive Care Unit (ICU). Coomey and Levison (1976) evaluated 62 children by comparing physical signs, subjective symptoms and pulmonary function studies (vide supra). While they found dyspnoea and auscultatory findings had no discriminant value, supraclavicular retraction and sternocleido-mastoid contraction were invariably associated with FVC, FEV_1 and maximal mid-expiratory flow rate (MEFR) values below 50% of predicted, indicative of severe disease. Pulsus paradoxus is also a sign of severely impaired lung function (vide supra). In a study of children aged 13 months to 15 years, Gallant et al (1978) found that increasing pulsus paradoxus correlated with worsening clinical scores. Pulsus paradoxus was significantly greater (mean 22 mmHg) in children with an arterial carbon dioxide tension above (compared with those below) 40 mmHg. The measurement of pulsus paradoxus by sphygmomanometry is difficult in the tachypnoeic, restless child with acute, severe asthma but it can be achieved. In the authors' experience, a useful clinical guide to pulsus paradoxus can be obtained by light palpation of the deep palmar arch. If the pulse can be felt to fade and return, pulsus paradoxus of greater than 20 mmHg is present, and is cause for immediate concern and admission to the ICU. Peak flow rates are unobtainable from infants and of marginal value for making decisions about ICU admission and therapy when acquired from acutely breathless older children.

ICU management of life-threatening asthma

The principles of therapy in this situation are similar to those presented earlier in this chapter. Nowadays, fewer asthmatic patients in this situation are seen in the ICU than in the past (in part, the result of better drugs and understanding of the disease by physician, patient and family). The corollary of this is that therapeutic interventions in the paediatric field are more often based on personal or anecdotal past experience, and adult or animal data, than on rigorous scientific studies involving numerous infants and children with life-threatening asthma. Our experience at the Children's Hospital of Los Angeles is based upon a steady 8-year background of 1000 admissions per year to the paediatric wards for acute asthma, with 25–30 infants and children per year being referred to the ICU. Of these, we intubate and mechanically ventilate from five to eight children per year. A few cautionary recommendations concerning monitoring, therapy and other interventions concerning the critically ill asthmatic are suggested.

Monitoring in the ICU

There is considerable variation throughout the world as to the quality of equipment and monitoring provided in paediatric ICUs. However, it is fundamental to the care of a critically ill asthmatic child who is in impending respiratory failure and being given intravenous and continuously nebulized drugs with potential major cardiac, respiratory, and neurological side effects, that appropriate monitoring be delivered. Heart rate and rhythm, respiratory waveform, arterial oxygen saturation, and plethysmographic trace should be continuously available and observable. Level of consciousness, fluid balance, colour, perfusion and temperature must be continually observed and recorded at close intervals. Transcutaneous carbon dioxide monitoring is useful, even in the paediatric patient, for continuous trend monitoring (Sivan et al, 1992).

Children with acute, severe asthma often require considerable blood sampling, particularly for serial serum electrolyte determinations, blood sugar determinations, and myocardial serum isoenzymes. Although arterial blood gases are not the sole determinant of therapeutic actions (vide infra), it is often useful to have direct determinations of pH, PaO_2, and $PaCO_2$. These values also help to 'calibrate' the range of tolerable SaO_2 and transcutaneous CO_2 values given by the indirect continuous monitoring methods. These needs, together with the continuous determination of blood pressure and pulsus paradoxus, along with the desire to minimize the discomfort of repeated percutaneous blood sampling for the patient, make a good case for the early installation of an arterial line. An anaesthetic and analgesic agent such as ketamine (vide infra) is useful to both the patient and the physician for this procedure.

Continuous intra-arterial blood gas electrodes are now commercially available. Unfortunately, in smaller children, these must be placed in the femoral rather than the radial artery. The systems are expensive and whether there are any significant long-term cost or management benefits from continuous blood gas sampling in asthma is yet to be determined. At this point, intermittent arterial blood gas sampling is sufficient, along with continuous oximetry and transcutaneous capnometry.

Once the patient is intubated, end-tidal carbon dioxide (CO_2) measurements are the best indirect, continuous evaluation of ventilation. It is important that both the value of end-tidal CO_2 tension and the waveform during inhalation and exhalation be displayed. The physiology associated with the measurements in severe $\dot{V}/\dot{Q}$ mismatch (as seen in life-threatening asthma), will ensure that prior to improvement, the end-tidal CO_2 value will sometimes be 10–15 mmHg lower than the corresponding arterial value (Sivan et al, 1992). The CO_2 trend and also the arterial-alveolar CO_2 difference will be helpful in managing both the ventilator and observing improvement in the disease. In addition, with obstructive airways disease the slope of the alveolar phase (as seen by capnography during exhalation) is always steep and will flatten as the disease improves.

As the ventilated asthmatic child improves, secretions are usually mobilized and these can contaminate both 'in-line' and 'side-stream' sampling techniques for CO_2. It is easy to see if such contamination has occurred, but it is more difficult to repair.

Supportive therapy

1. *Oxygen.* All patients with severe lower airway obstruction are hypoxaemic from $\dot{V}/\dot{Q}$ mismatching, and the degree of hypoxaemia correlates with the decline in forced expiratory flow. β-agonists delivered by any route can increase $\dot{V}/\dot{Q}$ mismatch and hence hypoxaemia. Humidified oxygen should be administered to maintain a PaO_2 above 60 mmHg (or SaO_2 above 90%). Oxygen at any concentration does not cause hypercapnia in the acute asthmatic attack in a child with no chronic pulmonary disease.

2. *Hydration.* Mild dehydration ($\leq 5\%$) is common in severe acute childhood asthma (Potter et al, 1991). Early correction of dehydration is always indicated, but excessive hydration may promote pulmonary fluid accumulation (Stalcup and Mellins, 1977) and will not loosen bronchial mucus plugs. Singleton et al (1986) have also shown that children with severe, acute asthma have impaired water excretion after water-loading and are at risk of hyponatraemia if given hypotonic fluids for a prolonged period of time. Isotonic, or only mildly hypotonic, intravenous fluid given at a rate of 50 ml/kg/24 hours appears safe and appropriate, after initial rehydration where necessary.

3. *Bicarbonate.* Metabolic acidosis is probably secondary to bicarbonate loss, under-utilization of lactate by hypoperfused liver and increased lactic acid production by respiratory muscles, especially when driven by β_2-agonists which increased oxygen consumption (Newth et al, 1991). In turn, acidosis has been reported to depress the myocardium and to limit the efficacy of β-agonists. We use bicarbonate to correct partially a metabolic acidosis (base excess ≤ -8) unresponsive to rehydration, and to buffer respiratory acidosis to a pH ≥ 7.25 when utilizing controlled hypoventilation in the intubated child.

4. *Sedatives.* These have been associated with respiratory depression and arrest in patients with acute, severe asthma. However, dyspnoea commonly promotes anxiety and can make for difficult management and therapy of a desperate young child in the paediatric ICU. In the ICU, where monitoring

is ideal, and expertise immediately available, an opportunity exists for using sedatives with direct bronchodilating properties. Ketamine is a dissociative anaesthetic with excellent analgesic and sedative properties. It is a useful agent for the placement of arterial lines for monitoring arterial blood gas (ABG) and blood pressure and it can be administered to both nonintubated and intubated asthmatic children. It possesses sympathomimetic actions and relaxes smooth muscle, with clinical improvement in peak inspiratory pressures, chest wall excursions, and arterial CO_2 tensions (Serma, 1992). Side effects of ketamine include arrhythmias due to catecholamine sensitization, an increase in secretions, and laryngospasm. We have used ketamine in doses from 3 to 10 mg/kg/hour for both intubated and nonintubated asthmatics for up to 5 days with no ill effects. We do administer a benzodiazepine in the form of midazolam at 1–4 μg/kg/minute to modify any possible emergence reactions.

5. *Antihistamines.* While there is no evidence these drugs worsen asthma, they have no proven value in the treatment of life-threatening asthma.

6. *Anticholinergic agents.* Atropine sulphate, atropine methonitrate, and ipratropium bromide are the most commonly available for bronchodilatation. In a few relatively small studies in children the concomitant use of inhaled ipratropium bromide and a selective β_2-agonist has been shown to produce a significant improvement in lung function compared with treatment with aerosolized β_2-agonist alone (Beck et al, 1985; Reisman et al, 1988). However, since completion of these studies, it is now unclear whether or not ipratropium has any added benefit in this situation (see earlier Section on Anticholinergic drugs).

7. *Aminophylline.* There has been considerable re-examination of the role of aminophylline in asthma (vide supra), but we continue to use it for life-threatening asthma in association with continuously nebulized or intravenous β-adrenoceptor agonists. Terbutaline (Jonkman et al, 1988) does not affect aminophylline kinetics, but the influence of salbutamol has not been examined; isoprenaline increases theophylline clearance (Hemstreet et al, 1982). Consequently, care must be taken in adjusting aminophylline administration, particularly when weaning down on intravenous isoprenaline, since serum concentrations of theophylline will tend to rise. Studies in patients and in dogs have indicated that no changes are seen in theophylline clearance due to mechanical ventilation (Hemstreet et al, 1982).

8. *β_2-adrenoceptor agonists.* Salbutamol (Katz et al, 1993) and terbutaline (Moler et al, 1988) have been used via continuous nebulization in children admitted to the ICU with status asthmaticus. We use full-strength solutions of both drugs, believing that the amount of drug which is delivered to the airways is dependent upon and limited by airflow obstruction. We have had no side effects with either drug apart from sinus tachycardia. Unfortunately, terbutaline as a chemical compound is only half as potent as salbutamol and

twice the amount must be administered to get the same bronchodilating effect. Since terbutaline is available in the United States only as a 1 mg/ml solution (compared with salbutamol at 5 mg/ml) there is a severe limitation on the therapeutic efficacy of this drug in the U.S. In other countries, where terbutaline is available as a 10 mg/ml respiratory solution, the drug should be as useful as salbutamol. We deliver salbutamol at up to 12.5 mg/kg/hour without ill effects. Selective β_2-adrenergic agonists do cause a decline in serum potassium by kaliuresis and increased intracellular uptake, so serum potassium must be monitored and corrected. A good aerosol delivery system is imperative when using continuously nebulized drugs, particularly when children are on positive-pressure ventilation and leaks are of paramount importance (Papo et al, 1993).

9. *Intravenous administration.* A review of our past 8 years' experience has shown that the use of full-strength, continuously nebulized salbutamol has neither decreased nor increased the length of ICU stay or complications for children admitted with status asthmaticus. However, a small proportion of children have not improved on continuously nebulized β-agonists, and have had progressive respiratory failure. Intravenous salbutamol, terbutaline, and isoprenaline may be used in these patients in an attempt to avoid mechanical ventilation, or to continue to treat bronchoconstriction when intervention with mechanical ventilation has become necessary. Myocardial ischaemia with ECG alteration, CPK-MB isoenzyme elevation and death have been associated with intravenous isoproterenol, but in the past 8 years of prospective evaluation and aggressive therapy, we have not had a death, nor have we seen enzyme or ECG evidence of myocardial ischaemia in asthmatics treated with this drug. While intravenous salbutamol (Bohn et al, 1984) and terbutaline (Fuglsang et al, 1989) have been shown to be effective in life-threatening asthma, we believe that isoprenaline retains a time-honoured and important role. For salbutamol and terbutaline, it is not clear from the literature what doses should be used. They have relatively long half-lives, and since doses are often increased slowly without intermittent boluses, it may take many hours for a new steady-state to be achieved, hence, the potential for underdosing is high. That notwithstanding, we have progressed to doses as high as 20 μg/kg/minute for terbutaline and 15 μg/kg/minute for salbutamol over time without ill effects. Isoprenaline has the advantage of having a very much shorter half-life (mean 4 minutes compared with 12 hours for terbutaline and salbutamol) (Hultquist et al, 1988; Reyes et al, 1993). Thus, side-effects such as tachycardia can, if necessary, quickly be controlled by turning off the infusion of isoprenaline. Clinical practice has shown that if the heart rate is kept between 190 and 200 beats per minute in an infant or child, there appears to be adequate delivery of the bronchodilator. Animal studies suggest tachyphylaxis to isoprenaline occurs with cardiac and skeletal muscle, but not with smooth muscle. Thus, the risk of underdosing with isoprenaline is theoretically minimized compared with salbutamol or terbutaline. Each time the heart rate drops below 180/minute, the infusion can be increased another 0.05 μg/kg/minute. We

have used progressive doses from 0.1 to 5.5 μg/kg/minute over hours, without ill effects.

10. *Magnesium sulphate.* There have been anecdotal reports of this drug alleviating asthma when given intravenously. The mechanism of action is not clear, though hypomagnesaemia has been reported in patients with bronchial asthma. To date, there have been no controlled studies on the use of magnesium sulphate in acute asthma in children. In cases where it is deemed necessary to try the drug, an intravenous infusion of 30–70 mg/kg over 20–30 minutes is the recommended dose.

11. *Inhalational agents.* Inhalational anaesthetic agents have been used sporadically for status asthmaticus unresponsive to maximal standard therapy. Unfortunately, many agents have serious side effects and in practice they are limited to intubated ventilated patients. Halogen hydrocarbons have been implicated in severe hepatic and renal toxicity. While halothane and enflurane are not directly toxic, their metabolic products appear to be responsible for a rare form of hepatic necrosis. Isofluorane, a halogenated ether is an anaesthetic agent that produces bronchodilatation through a number of mechanisms (Johnson et al, 1990). Isofluorane undergoes minimal metabolism and, to our knowledge, there are no documented cases of isofluorane-induced hepatic or renal injury. Scavenging exhaust gases in the ICU is necessary to prevent long-term anaesthetic exposure for health-care personnel. Suitable equipment is usually simple and inexpensive.

12. *Intubation and mechanical ventilation.* The indications for intubation and mechanical ventilation in paediatric patients with severe asthma are, by and large, arbitrary. The only absolute indications for intubation and mechanical ventilation are a decreased level of consciousness and near-complete or complete apnoea. Other possible indications include evidence of compromized organ perfusion such as hypotension, decreased urinary output, progressive metabolic acidosis, severe cardiac arrhythmias, pneumothorax, and a steadily decreasing PaO_2 (less than 60 mmHg unrelieved by oxygen) and/or increasing $PaCO_2$ despite maximal pharmacological therapy. Traditionally, much attention has been focused on the importance of hypercapnia as a predictor of those requiring both intensive care and ventilation. In the early 1970s, a subsequently popular asthma score was devised (Downes et al, 1973) which was heavily weighted by a rising arterial carbon dioxide tension. However, at this time there must be serious reservations about the applicability of the so-called Wood–Downes criteria (Downes et al, 1973). Mountain and Sahn (1988) reported in adult asthmatic patients that mechanical ventilation was required in only 8% of 61 episodes of hypercapnia accompanying acute asthma. Current management, therefore, dictates that arterial blood gases alone are inadequate for decision making. On some occasions it is entirely appropriate to manage patients without ventilation even with a high arterial CO_2 tension, provided some therapeutic options are yet to be instituted. Conversely, there are other occasions when a patient is obviously failing clinically, even when

the arterial CO_2 tension is relatively low, or when it is still quite low but rising despite maximal therapy having been instituted.

Reviews of severe, acute asthma suggest that up to 33% of children admitted to a paediatric ICU will require mechanically assisted ventilation, and up to 8% of them will die (Stein et al, 1989). Historically, fear of the consequences of mechanical ventilation has been justified. Previous generations of ventilators delivered mandatory, preset tidal volumes regardless of the dynamics of the respiratory system, with enormous potential for gas-trapping, dynamic hyperinflation, and subsequent pulmonary barotrauma and circulatory depression. The development of time-cycled, pressure-limited ventilators represented a substantial advance in this field. The strategy of (pressure) controlled hypoventilation as a means of limiting complications was originally proposed in 1984 (Darioli and Perret, 1984). Subsequently, it has been embraced in paediatric practice and both good experience and outcomes have been reported (Dworkin and Katta, 1989; Cox et al, 1991). While this approach of 'permissive hypercapnia' has been recently endorsed by a consensus conference on mechanical ventilation (Slutsky, 1994), the exact levels to which arterial CO_2 should be permitted to rise and pH to fall have yet to be determined. However, $PaCO_2$ levels of 90–150 mmHg and a pH of 7.00 or more appear to be safe, especially if these levels are achieved gradually and without hypoxaemia (Goldstein et al, 1990).

In most paediatric ICUs, uncuffed endotracheal tubes are routinely used in infants and children under 8 years of age to minimize laryngeal injury, while cuffed tubes are used in older children. However, air leakage can cause significant difficulties during assisted ventilation of children with increased airways resistance and decreased pulmonary compliance. In such cases, intubation with a cuffed endotracheal tube is indicated, and it has been shown recently that even in small children the use of modern high-volume, low-pressure cuffed tubes is not associated with higher rates of either early or late subglottic complications when careful tube care and size selection are employed (Deakers et al, 1994).

13. *Neuromuscular blockade and corticosteroids.* Competitive inhibitor blocking agents such as pancuronium and vecuronium are frequently used in ventilated infants and children. Indications for their use include insufficient sedation to control the child's agitation and combativeness, inefficient ventilation, and high airways resistance with low lung compliance—all conditions which are common in severe, acute asthma. In recent years, several reports have raised the issue of prolonged neuromuscular weakness and even paralysis after a few days of neuromuscular relaxant administration (Segredo et al, 1992). Two patterns of neuromuscular dysfunction secondary to the use of muscle relaxants have been reported. One is persistent neuromuscular junction blockade secondary to accumulation of the drug or one of its metabolites most commonly observed in patients with renal failure. The second pattern is poorly understood and is attributed to generalized myopathy with histopathological findings of atrophy, necrosis, and degeneration of muscle fibres. This pattern has been associated with

prolonged use of neuromuscular blocking agents, especially with the con-comitant use of corticosteroids (Hansen–Flaschen et al, 1993). Recovery from this type of neuromuscular dysfunction may take weeks or months. This association presents a major problem for children mechanically venti-lated for acute asthma. While we have seen this neuromuscular compli-cation, its incidence in children may be lower than in adult asthmatic patients. At this juncture, neuromuscular blockade should be used for as short a time as possible for ventilated asthmatic children, with considerable reliance on heavy sedation to achieve ventilator-patient synchronization. In addition, it may be that nonsteroid-like neuromuscular blocking agents such as atracurium and doxacurium should be used in case the steroidal structures of pancuronium and vecuronium (and some of their metabolites) somehow contribute synergistically to an adverse effect on skeletal muscle.

Fatal or near-fatal asthma

A number of investigators have studied near-fatal attacks in an endeavour to understand the pathophysiology of severe or catastrophic asthma. Molfino and Slutsky (1994) reviewed the literature in this area and attempted to identify both the risk and precipitating factors. Severe attacks can occur even when there are no identifiable risk factors. O'Hollaran et al (1991) demonstrated that many of these episodes were seasonally clustered and suggested that the near-fatal attacks may have been triggered by exposure to an aero-allergen. Roux and Weinberger (1993) found a similar seasonal pattern in children with near-fatal asthma. Arnold et al (1982) identified a group of patients in whom rapid and overwhelming deteriora-tion of asthma can occur. Sampson et al (1992) examined the role of food allergy in triggering fatal and near-fatal episodes of asthma in children. The role of β_2-adrenergic agonist drugs in the causation of deaths from asthma remains uncertain (Warner, 1994). Sur et al (1993) reported histological differences in the airway inflammation in sudden onset fatal asthma and speculated that it was a distinct entity with few eosinophils and more neutrophils in the airway submucosa. Kiruchi et al (1994) reported reduced chemosensitivity to hypoxia and blunted perception to dyspnoea in patients with a near-fatal attack of asthma.

It has been recognized that the inability of the patient or physician to recognize asthma severity is a major contributing factor to fatal and near-fatal episodes (Stableforth, 1987). This in turn may bear on the statistic that asthmatic patients in the ICU have a lower mortality than those admitted initially to general hospital wards, although the latter may be assumed less severely ill on admission. The rapid deterioration in pulmonary function, characteristic of the patients who die from asthma, is probably recognized and treated earlier in the ICU setting.

After the crisis is over

There are no absolute criteria for discharge from hospital. As with the initial decision to admit the patient, this decision will be influenced by a range of medical and social factors. The International Consensus Report (1992) recommends the following criteria for discharge from hospital:

(i) short-acting inhaled β_2-adrenergic agonist is needed no more than every 4 hours;
(ii) patient is not waking at night or in the early morning requiring bronchodilator;
(iii) clinical examination is normal or near normal;
(iv) PEF or FEV_1 is > 70–80% of that predicted;
(v) patient is able to use inhaler devices correctly;
(vi) patient's previous Asthma Management Plan is reviewed and modified if necessary;
(vii) appropriate arrangements for follow-up have been made.

These criteria may be varied according to the physician's knowledge of the individual patient and their family.

SUMMARY

The chapter reviews information in three main areas related to the treatment of acute asthma in children: drug delivery to the respiratory tract, cellular and clinical pharmacology of asthma medications and the recognition and treatment of acute asthma in children.

Successful delivery of medication to the respiratory tract is central to the successful treatment of asthma. The particular problems associated with medication delivery to young children are reviewed and recommendations made regarding age-appropriate delivery devices.

The cellular and clinical pharmacology of the wide range of medications used in the treatment of acute asthma is reviewed. Recent developments in receptor pharmacology and the mechanism of action of bronchodilators and corticosteroids are reviewed in detail.

A structured approach to the recognition and treatment of acute asthma in children is provided with specific emphasis on assessing the severity of asthma and assigning appropriate therapy. The management of the child at home, in hospital and in intensive care is reviewed.

APPENDIX

Asthma medical history checklist

1. Nature of symptoms
Cough, wheeze, chest tightness, exercise related symptoms

2. Pattern of symptoms
Year round, specific seasons, change of season
Continuous or episodic
Onset, duration and frequency of symptoms
Nocturnal asthma

3. *Precipitating or aggravating factors*
   Viral respiratory infections (is child in day-care?)
   Weather changes, cool air, environmental changes
   Exposure to irritants, e.g. cigarette smoke
   Exercise-induced asthma
   Exposure to known allergens
   Food additives—colourings, meta-bisulphite, monosodium glutamate
   Food (food allergies, especially to dairy products, are uncommon cause of asthma in children)
   Exposure to chemicals or irritants in the work-place or at home
   Nature of dwelling

4. *Past history*
   Age of onset, age at diagnosis
   Progress of disease over time (better or worse)
   Previous treatments and responses
   Frequency of symptoms
   Frequency of exacerbations
   History of emergency room visits and admissions
   History of life-threatening attacks and ICU admissions
   Limitation of physical activity

5. *Current management*
   Current medications
   Current symptom control

6. *Profile of typical exacerbation*
   Usual trigger
   Usual time course, especially the amount of time between first signs or symptoms and subsequent
       deterioration.
   Current Asthma Management Plan
   Usual outcome and duration

7. *Home environment*
   Pets, smoking and other factors

8. *Impact of disease*
   Time off school/work
   Limitation of physical activity
   Sleep disturbance due to nocturnal asthma
   Effects of disease or medication on growth
   Impact on family functioning

9. *Assessment of patient/parent knowledge about medications and Asthma Management Plan*

10. *Family history of asthma and related atopic disorders*

11. *General health and other prescribed medications*
    Inquire specifically about medications known to aggravate
    asthma, e.g. β-blockers for hypertension or glaucoma
    aspirin and nonsteroidal anti-inflammatory drugs

REFERENCES

Agertoft L & Pedersen S (1993) Importance of the inhalation device on the effect of budesonide. *Archives of Diseases in Childhood* **69**: 130–133.

Anderson GP, Linden A & Rabe K (1994) Why are long-acting beta-adrenoceptor agonists long-acting? *European Respiratory Journal* **7**: 569–579.

Arnold AG, Lane DJ & Zapata E (1982) The speed of onset and severity of acute asthma. British Journal of *Diseases of the Chest* **76**: 157–163.

Asthma Management Handbook (1993) Melbourne: National Asthma Campaign.

Aubier M, De Troyer A, Sampson M et al (1981) Aminophylline improves diaphragmatic contractility. *New England Journal of Medicine* **305**: 249–252.

Bai TR, Mak JC & Barnes PJ (1992) A comparison of beta-adrenergic receptors and in vitro relaxant responses to isoproterenol in asthmatic airway smooth muscle. *American Journal of Respiratory, Cellular & Molecular Biology* **6**: 647–651.

Barnes NC (1992) Effects of corticosteroids in acute severe asthma. *Thorax* **47**: 582–583.

Barnes PJ (1991) Anticholinergics in COPD: Theoretical implications. *Pathway to Successful Management Part I. Research and Clinical Forums* **13**: 33–42.

Barnes PJ (1993) Theoretical aspects of anticholinergic treatment. In Gross NJ (ed.) *Anticholinergic Therapy in Obstructive Airway Disease*, pp 88–104. London: Franklin Scientific Publications.

Barnes PJ & Lee KH (1992) Recent advances in asthma. *Postgradnase Medical Journal 68:* 942–953.

Barnes P & Adcock I (1993) Anti-inflammatory actions of steroids: molecular mechanisms of action. *Trends in Phamacologic Science* **14**: 436–441.

Barnes PJ & Pauwels R. (1994) Theophylline in the management of asthma: time for reappraisal? *European Respiratory Journal* **7**: 579–591.

Batty KT, Gardiner FS & Kendall PA (1994) Asthma knowledge in acute severe asthma. *Medical Journal of Australia* **160**: 609–610.

Bauer R & Banholzer R (1993) Pharmacology of quaternary anti-cholinergic drugs in asthma – In Gross NJ (ed.) *Anticholinergic Therapy in Obstructive Airway Disease*, pp 105–115. London: Franklin Scientific Publications.

Beasley R, Pearce N, Crane J et al (1991) Asthma mortality and inhaled beta-agonist therapy. *Australia and New Zealand Journal of Medicine* **21**: 753–763.

Beck R, Robertson C, Galdes–Sebaldt M & Levison H (1985) Combined salbutamol and ipratropium bromide by inhalation in the treatment of severe acute asthma. *Journal of Pediatrics* **107**: 605–608.

Beer S, Laver J, Karpuch J et al (1987) Prodromal features of asthma. *Archives of Disease in Childhood* **62**: 345–348.

Bergstrand H (1980) Phosphodiesterase inhibition and theophylline. *European Journal of Respiratory Disease* **1 (supplement 109)**: 37–44.

Bisgaard H (1993) Dose of aerosol inhaled by young children from a small-volume spacer (Baby-spacer) (Abstract). *European Journal Respiratory Disease* **6 (supplement 17)**: 352.

Bisgaard H (1994) Aerosol treatment of young children. *European Respiratory Review* **4**: 15–20.

Bohn D, Kalloghlian A, Jenkins J et al (1984) Intravenous salbutamol in the treatment of status asthmaticus in children. *Critical Care Medicine* **12**: 892–896.

Bollinger C, Fourie P, Kotze D & Joubert J (1992) Relation of measures of asthma severity and response to treatment to outcome in severe acute asthma. *Thorax* **47**: 943–947.

Bone RC & Burch SG (1991) Management of status asthmaticus. *Annals of Allergy* **67**: 461–469.

Boner A, Piacentini G & Bellanti J (1993) The need for early interventions in childhood asthma. *Annals of Allergy* **71**: 85–94.

Bowler SD, Mitchell CA & Armstrong JG (1987) Nebulised fenoterol and intravenous aminophylline in acute severe asthma. *European Journal of Respiratory Disease* **70**: 280–283.

Bowler SD, Mitchell CA & Armstrong JG (1992) Corticosteroids in acute severe asthma: effectiveness of low doses. *Thorax* **47**: 584–587.

Brattsand R (1992) Glucocorticoid steroids: molecular mechanism of action. *American Review of Respiratory Disease.* **146**: S1360–S1361.

British Thoracic Society (1993) Guidelines on the management of asthma *Thorax* **48 (supplement)**: S1–S24.

Canny G, Reisman J, Healy R et al (1989) Acute Asthma: Observations regarding the treatment in a paediatric emergency room. *Pediatrics* **83**: 507–512.

Carmen PG & Landau L (1990) Increased paediatric admissions with asthma in Western Australia— a problem of diagnosis? *Medical Journal of Australia* **152**: 23–26.

Carter E, Cruz M, Chesrown S et al (1993) Efficacy of intravenously administered theophylline in children hospitalised with severe asthma. *Journal of Pediatrics* **122**: 470–476.

Cerrina J, Ladivric LR, Labat B et al (1986) Comparison of human bronchial muscle responses to histamine in vivo with histamine and isoproterenol agonists in vitro. *American Review of Respiratory Disease* **134**: 57–61.

Clarke J, Aston H & Silverman M (1993) Delivery of salbutamol by metered dose inhaler and valved spacer to wheezy infants: effect on bronchial responsiveness. *Archives of Disease in Childhood* **69**: 125–129.

Collis G, Cole C & Le Souef P (1990) Dilution of nebulised aerosols by entrainment in children. *Lancet* **336:** 341–343.

Conway SP & Littlewood JM (1985) Admission to hospital with asthma. *Archives of Disease in Childhood* **60:** 636–639.

Conner WT, Dolovich M, Frame R, & Newhouse M (1989) Reliable salbutamol administration in 3- to 36 month-old children by means of a metered dose inhaler and Aerochamber with mask. *Pediatric Pulmonology* **6:** 263–267.

Coomey J & Levison H (1976) Physical signs in childhood asthma. *Pediatrics* **61:** 46–51.

Connett GJ, Warde C, Wooler E & Lenney W (1993) Prednisolone and salbutamol in the hospital treatment of acute asthma. *Archives of Disease in Childhood* **70:** 170–173.

Connett G & Lenney W (1993) Prevention of viral induced asthma attacks using inhaled budesonide. *Archives of Disease in Childhood* **68:** 85–87.

Cox RG, Barker GA & Bohn DJ (1991) Efficacy, results, and complications of mechanical ventilation in children with status asthmaticus. *Pediatric Pulmonology* **11:** 120–126.

Cypar D & Busse W (1993) Steroid resistant asthma. *Journal of Allergy and Clinical Immunology* **92:** 362–372.

Darioli R & Perret C (1984) Mechanical controlled hypoventilation in status asthmaticus. *American Review of Respiratory Disease* **129:** 385–387.

Davis A, Vickerson F, Worsley G et al (1984) Determination of dose-response relationship for ipratropium bromide in asthmatic children. *Journal of Pediatrics* **105:** 1002–1005.

Deakers TW, Reynolds G, Stretton M & Newth CJ (1994) Cuffed endotracheal tubes in pediatric intensive care. *Journal of Pediatrics* **125:** 57–62.

Derom E, Joos G, Kips J et al (1994) Factors influencing pulmonary absorption of inhaled drugs. *European Respiratory Review* **4:** 71–74.

Di Guilio GA, Kercsmar CM, King SE et al (1993) Hospital treatment of acute asthma: lack of benefit from theophylline given in addition to nebulized albuterol and intravenously administered corticosteroid. *Journal of Pediatrics* **122:** 464–469.

Dolan LM, Kesarwala H & Holroyde JC (1987) Short-term high-dose systemic steroids in children with acute asthma: the effect on the hypo-thalamic-pituitary-adrenal axis. *Journal of Allergy and Clinical Immunology* **80:** 81–87.

Dolovich M & Newhouse M (1993) Aerosols: generation, methods of administration, and therapeutic applications in asthma. In Middleton E, Reed C, Ellis E et al (eds) *Allergy: Principles and Practice*, pp 712–739. St Louis; CV Mosby.

Downes JJ, Wood DW, Harwood I et al (1973) Intravenous isoproterenol infusion in children with severe hypercapnia due to status asthmaticus. Effects on ventilation, circulation, and clinical scores. *Critical Care Medicine* **1:** 63–78.

DuPlooy WJ, Hay L, Kahler CP et al (1994) The dose related hyper and hypokalaemic effects of salbutamol and its arrhythmogenic potential. *British Journal of Pharmacology* **111:** 73–76.

Dworkin G & Kattan M (1989) Mechanical ventilation for status asthmaticus in children. *Journal of Pediatrics* **114:** 545–549.

Estenne M, Yernault J & DeTroyer A (1980) Effects of parenteral aminophylline on lung mechanics in normal humans. *American Review of Respiratory Disease* **121:** 967–971.

Fuglsang G, Pedersen S & Borgström L (1989) Dose-response relationships of intravenously administered terbutaline in children with asthma. *Journal of Pediatrics* **114:** 315–320.

Fraser CM, Nelson HS & Middleton E (1993) Adrenergic agonists. In Middleton E, Reed C, Ellis E et al (eds) *Allergy; Principles and Practice*, 4th edn, pp. 778–784. St. Louis: CV Mosby.

Gallant ST, Groncy CE & Shaw KC (1978) The value of pulsus paradoxus in assessing a child with status asthmaticus. *Pediatrics* **61:** 46–51.

Geelhoed GC (1988) Predictive value of oxygen saturation in emergency evaluation of asthmatic children. *Bristish Medical Journal* **297:** 395–396.

Gershel J, Golman H, Stein R et al (1983) The usefulness of chest radiographs in first asthma attacks. *New England Journal of Medicine* **309:** 336–339.

Goldie RG, Spina D, Henry P et al (1986) In vitro responsiveness of human asthmatic bronchus to carbachol, histamine, beta-adrenoreceptor agonists and theophylline. *British Journal of Clinical Pharmacology* **22:** 669–676.

Goldstein B, Shannon DC & Todres ID (1990) Supercarbia in children: clinical course and outcome. *Critical Care Medicine* **18:** 166–168.

Grace RF (1994) Pulse oximetry: gold standard or false sense of security. *Medical Journal of Austrialia* **160:** 638–644.

Greening AP, Ind PW, Northfield M & Shaw G (1994) Added salmeterol versus higher-dose corticosteroid in patients with symptoms on existing inhaled steroid. *Lancet* **344:** 219–224.

Gross NJ (1988) Ipratropium bromide. *New England Journal of Medicine* **319:** 486–494.

Gross NJ (1993) Safety and side-effects of anti-cholinergic bronchodilators. In Gross NJ (ed.) *Anticholinergic Therapy in Obstructivea Airway Disease*, pp 116–127. London: Franklin Scientific Publications.

Guidelines for Diagnosis and Managment of Asthma (1991) Betreseda: National Institutes of Health.

Hansen–Flaschen J, Cowen J & Raps EC (1993) Neuromuscular blockade in the intensive care unit. More than we bargained for. *American Review of Respiratory Disease* **147:** 234–236.

Hardy J, Newman S & Knoch M (1993) Lung deposition from four nebulisers. *Respiratory Medicine* **87:** 451–465.

Hemstreet MP, Miles MV & Rutland RO (1982) Effective intravenous isoproterenol on theophylline kinetics. *Journal of Allergy and Clinical Immunology* **69:** 361–364.

Hendeles L, Weinberger M & Szefler S (1992) Safety and efficacy of theophylline in children with asthma. *Journal of Pediatrics* **120:** 177–183.

Henry R (1990) Ipratropium bromide: An additive effect? *Journal of Pediatrics and Child Health* **26:** 124–125.

Henry R, Robertson C, Asher I et al (1993) Consensus view: Management of acute asthma. *Journal of Pediatrics and Child Health* **29:** 101–103.

Hill MR, Szettler SJ, Ball BD et al (1990) Monitoring glucocorticoid therapy: a pharmacokinetic approach. *Clinical Pharacology and Therapy* **48:** 390–398.

Ho L, Landau LI & Le Souef PN (1994) Lack of efficacy of single dose prednisolone in moderately severe asthma. *Medical Journal of Australia* **160:** 701–704.

Hofmann W, Maroten T & Graham R (1989) Predicted deposition of nonhydroscopic aerosols in the human lung as a function of subject age. *Journal of Aerosol Medicine* **2:** 49–68.

Hultquist C, Lindberg C, Nyberg L et al (1989) Pharmacokinetics of intravenous terbutaline in asthmatic children. *Development Pharmacology Therapeutics* **13:** 11–20.

Hyndman SJ, Williams DR, Merrill SL et al (1994) Rates of admission to hospital for asthma. *British Medical Journal* **308:** 1596–1600.

Idris A, McDermott M, Raucci J et al (1993) Emergency Department of severe asthma: metered dose inhaler plus holding chamber is equivalent in effectiveness to nebuliser. *Chest* **103:** 655–672.

International Consensus Report on Diagnosis and Treatment of Asthma (1992) National Heart, Lung and Blood Institute, National Institutes of Health, Bethesda.

Isles AF & Newth CJL (1993) The wheezing infant. In. Schatz M & Zeiger RS (eds) *Asthma and Allergy in Pregancy and Early Infancy*, pp 503–533. New York: Marcel Dekker.

Jenkins CR & Woolcock AJ (1988) Effect of prednisone and beclomethasone diproprionate on airway responsiveness in asthma: a comparative study. *Thorax* **43:** 378–390.

Jenne J (1994) What role for theophylline? (Editorial) *Thorax* **49:** 97–100.

Johnson M (1992) Salmeterol: a novel drug for the treatment of asthma. In Anderson GP & Morley J (eds) *New Drugs for Asthma*, pp 79–95 Basel: Birkhauser Verlag.

Johnson RG, Noseworthy TW, Friesen EG et al (1990) Isoflurane therapy for status asthmaticus in children in adults. *Chest* **97:** 698–701.

Jones TR, Chorette L, Garcia ML & Kaczorowski GJ (1990) Selective inhibition of relaxation of guinea-pig trachea by charybodotoxin, a potent calcium activated K-channel inhibitor. *Journal of Pharmacology and Experimented Therapy* **225:** 697–706.

Jonkman JH, Borgstrom L, van der Boon WJ & de Noord OE (1988) Theophylline-terbutaline, a steady state study on possible pharmacokinetic interactions with special reference to chronopharmacokinetic aspects. *British Journal of Clinical Pharmacology* **26:** 285–293.

Kamada AK, Leung DY & Szefler SJ (1992) Steroid resistance in asthma: our current understanding. *Pediatric Pulmonology* **14:** 180–186.

Kamada AK, Spahn JD, Surs W et al (1994) Coexistence of glucocorticoreceptor and pharmacokinetic abnormalities: factors that contribute to a poor response to treatment with glucocorticoids in children with asthma. *Journal of Pediatrics* **124:** 984–986.

Katz RW, Kelly HW, Crowley MR et al (1993) Safety of continuous nebulized albuterol for bronchospasm in infants and children. *Pediatrics* **92:** 666–669.

Kerem E, Levison H, Schuh S et al (1993) Efficacy of albuterol administered by nebuliser versus spacer device in children with acute asthma. *Journal of Pediatrics* **123:** 313–317.

Kiruchi Y, Okabe S, Tamura G et al (1994) Chemosensitivity and perception of dyspnoea in patients with a history of near-fatal asthma. *New England Journal of Medicine* **330:** 1329–1334.

Kraemer R, Frey U, Sommer C & Russi E (1991) Short-term effect of albuterol delivered by a new auxiliary device in wheezy infants. *American Review of Respiratory Disease* **144:** 347–351.

Kun HY, Oates RK & Mellis CM (1993) Hospital admissions and attendances for asthma—a true increase? *Medical Journal of Australia* **159:** 312–313.

Littenberg B & Gluck E (1986) A controlled trial of methylprednisolone in the emergency treatment of acute asthma. *New England Journal of Medicine* **314:** 150–152.

Lundgen JD, Kaliner MA & Shelhamer JH (1990) Mechanisms by which glucocorticosteroids inhibit secretion of mucus in asthmatic airways. *American Review of Respiratory Disease* **141:** S52–58.

Mann JS & Holgate ST (1985) Specific antagonism of adenosine induced bronchoconstriction in asthma by oral theophylline. *British Journal of Clinical Pharmacology* **19:** 85–92.

Maxham J (1988) Aminophylline and respiratory muscles: an alternative view. *Clinical Chest Medicine* **12:** 325–340.

McFadden ER (1994a) Management of patients with acute asthma: what do we know? What do we need to know? *Annals of Allergy* **72:** 385–389.

McFadden ER (1994b) Are there risks associated with beta-agonists? The data reviewed. *International Respiratory Forum* **1:** 27–33.

Miesfeld RL (1990) Molecular mechanisms of corticosteroid action. *American Review of Respiratory Disease* **141:** S11–17.

Mitenko P & Ogilvie R (1973) Rational intravenous doses of theophylline. *New England Journal of Medicine* **289:** 85–92.

Moler FW, Herwitz ME & Custer JR (1988) Improvement in clinical asthma score and $PaCO_2$ in children with severe asthma treated with continuously nebulized terbutaline. *Journal of Allergy and Clinical Immunology* **81:** 1101–1109.

Molfino NA & Slutsky AS (1994) Near-fatal asthma. *European Respiratory Journal* **7:** 981–990.

Morley J, Sanjar S & Newth CJL (1990) Viewpoint: Untoward effects of beta-adrenoceptor agonists in asthma. *European Respiratory Journal* **3:** 228–237.

Mountain R & Sahn S (1988) Clinical features and outcome in patients with acute asthma representing with hypercapnia. *American Review of Respiratory Disease* **138:** 535–539.

Mullen M, Mullen B & Cavey C (1993) The association between beta-agonist use and death from asthma: a meta-analytic integration of case-control studies. *Journal of the American Medical Association* **270:** 1842–1845.

Munch A, Medel DB, Smith LI & Orti E (1990) Glucocorticoid receptors and actions. *American Review of Respiratory Disease* **141:** S2–10.

Murphy S & Kelly H (1991) Management of acute asthma. *Pediatrician* **18:** 287–300.

Naspitz CK & Sole D (1992) Treatment of acute wheezing and dyspnoea attacks in children under 2 years old: Inhalation of fenoterol plus ipratropium bromide versus fenoterol. *Journal of Asthma* **29:** 253–258.

Newman S & Pavia D (1985) Aerosol deposition in man. In Moren F, Newhouse M & Dolovich M (eds) *Aerosols in Medicine*, pp 193–217 Amsterdam; Elsevier.

Newman SP (1991) Aerosol generators and delivery systems. *Respiratory Care* **36:** 939–951.

Newth CJL, Amsler B, Anderson G & Morley J (1991) The ventilatory and oxygen costs in the anesthetised Rhesus monkey of inhaling drugs used in the therapy and diagnosis of asthma. *American Review of Respiratory Disease* **143:** 766–771.

Oberklaid F, Mellis CM, Le Souef P et al (1993) A comparison of a body-weight dose versus a fixed dose of nebulised salbutamol in acute asthma in children. *Medical Journal of Australia* **158:** 751–753.

O'Callaghan C (1993) How to get drugs into the respiratory tract. *Archives of Disease in Childhood* **68:** 441–443.

O'Hollaren MT, Yunginger JW, Offord KP et al (1991) Exposure to aeroallergen as a possible precipitating factor in respiratory arrest in young patients with asthma. *New England Journal of Medicine* **324:** 359–363.

Papo MC, Frank J & Thompson AE (1993) A prospective randomized study of continuous versus intimate nebulized albuterol for severe status asthmaticus in children. *Critical Care Medicine* **21:** 1479–1486.

Pauwels R & Persson C (1991) Xanthines. In Kaliner MA, Barnes PJ & Persson CG (eds) *Asthma: its Pathology and Treatment*, pp 503–519. New York: Marcel Dekker.

Peat JK, van den Berg RH, Green WF et al (1994) Changing prevalence of asthma in Australian children. *British Medical Journal* **308:** 1591–1596.

Pedersen S, Frost L & Arnfred T (1986) Errors in inhalation technique and efficacy in inhaler use in asthmatic children. *Allergy* **41:** 118–124.

Pedersen S, Hansen OR & Fugslang G (1990) Influence of inspiratory flow rate upon the effect of a Turbuhaler. *Archives of Disease in Childhood* **65:** 308–319.

Pedersen (1994) Choice of inhalation therapy in paediatrics. *European Respiratory Review* **4:** 85–88.

Permutt S (1973) Physiologic changes in the acute asthma attack. In Austen K & Lichenstein LM (eds) *Asthma: Physiology, Immunopharmacology, and Treatment* pp 15–24. New York: Academic Press.

Phalen R, Oldham M, Kleinman M & Crocker T (1988) Tracheobronchial deposition characteristics for infants, children and adolescents. *Annals of Occupational Hygienic* **33 (supplement):** 11–21.

Phelan P (1992) Childhood asthma: the role of corticosteroids. *Modern Medicine (Australia)* Aug: 11–14.

Potter PC, Klein M & Weinberg EG (1991) Hydration in severe acute asthma. *Archives of Disease in Childhood* **66:** 216–219.

Reisman J, Galdes-Sebaldt M, Kazim F et al (1988) Frequent administration by inhalation of salbutamol and ipratropium bromide in the initial management of severe acute asthma in children. *Journal of Allergy and Clinical Immunology* **81:** 16–20.

Reisman J, Canney G & Levison H (1993) The role of anti-cholinergic drugs in paediatric airway disease. In Gross NJ (ed.) *Anticholinergic Therapy in Obstructive Airway Disease*, pp 169–180. London: Franklin Scientific Publications.

Reyes G, Schwartz PH, Newth CJ & Eldadah MK (1993) The pharmacokinetics of isoproterenol on critically ill pediatric patients. *Journal of Clinical Pharmacology* **32:** 29–34.

Robertson CF, Smith F, Beck R, & Levison H (1985) Response to frequent low doses of nebulized salbutamol in acute asthma. *Journal of Pediatrics* **106:** 672–674.

Robertson CF, Heycock E, Bishop J et al (1991) Prevalence of asthma in Melbourne schoolchildren: changes over 26 years. *British Medical Journal* **302:** 1116–1118.

Robertson CF, Rubinfeld A & Bowes G (1992) Paediatric asthma deaths in Victoria. *Pediatric Pulmonology* **13:** 95–100.

Roux P & Weinberger EG (1993) Seasonal and recurrent intensive care admission for acute severe asthma in children. *South African Medical Journal* **83:** 177–179.

Salmeron S, Brochard L, Mal H et al (1994) Nebulized -v-intravenous albuterol in hypercapnic acute asthma. *American Journal of Respiratory and Critical Care Medicine* **149:** 1466–1470.

Sampson HA, Mendelson L & Rosen JP (1992) Fatal and near-fatal anaphylactic reactions to food in children and adolescents. *New England Journal of Medicine* **327:** 380–384.

Schuh S, Parkin P & Rajan A (1989) High versus low-dose nebulized albuterol in children with acute severe asthma. *Pediatrics* **83:** 513–518.

Schuh S, Reider M, Canny G et al (1990) Nebulized albuterol in acute childhood asthma: Comparison of two doses. *Pediatrics* **86:** 509–513.

Sears MR (1987) Are deaths from asthma really on the rise? *Journal of Respiratory Disease* **8:** 39–49.

Segredo B, Coldwell JD, Matthay MA et al (1992) Persistent paralysis in critically ill patients after long-term administration of vecuronium. *New England Journal of Medicine* **327:** 524.

Serma VJ (1992) Use of ketamine in acute severe asthma. *Acta Anaesthesiologica Scandinavica* **36:** 106–107.

Sheffer AL (1991) Guidelines for the diagnosis and management of asthma VIII: Acute exacerbations of asthma. *Journal of Allergy and Clinical Immunology* **88:** 493–518.

Shlermer RP (1990) Effect of glucocorticoids on inflammatory cells relevant to their therapeutic application in asthma. *American Review of Respiratory Disease* **141:** S39–43.

Silverman M (1990) Aerosol therapy in the newborn. *Archives of Disease in childhood* **64:** 1270–1273.

Singh M & Kumar L (1993) Continuous nebulised salbutamol plus oral once a day prednisolone in status asthmaticus. *Archives of Disease in Childhood* **69:** 416–419.

Singleton R, Moel D & Cohn R (1986) Preliminary observations of impaired water excretion in treated status asthmaticus. *American Journal of Diseases in Children* **140:** 59–61.

Sivan Y, Eldadah MK, Cheah T & Newth CJL (1992) Estimation of arterial carbon dioxide by end-tidal and transcutaneous PCO_2 measurements in ventilated children. *Pediatric Pulmonology* **12:** 153–157.

Slutsky AS (1994) Consensus conference on mechanical ventilation. *Intensive Care Medicine* **20:** 64–79.

Sly P, Cahill P, Willet K & Burton P (1994) Accuracy of mini-peak flow meters in indicating changes in lung function in children with asthma. *British Medical Journal* **308:** 572–574.

Small RC, Chiu P, Cook SJ et al (1993) Beta-adrenoceptor agonists in bronchial asthma: role of potassium channel opening in mediating their bronchodilator effects. *Clinical Experimental Allergy* **23:** 802–811.

Stableforth DE (1987) Asthma mortality and physician competence. *Journal of Allergy and Clinical Immunology* **80::** 463–466.

Stalcup SA & Mellins RB (1977) Mechanical forces producing pulmonary edema in acute asthma. *New England Journal of Medicine* **297:** 592–596.

Stein R, Canny GJ, Bohn DJ et al (1989) Severe acute asthma in a pediatric intensive care unit: six years' experience. *Pediatrics* **83:** 1023–1028.

Stempel D & Redding G (1992) Management of acute asthma. *Pediatric Clinics of North America* **39:** 1311–1325.

Sterk PJ (1994) Are there risks associated with beta-agonists? A physiologic perspective. *International Respiratory Forum* **1:** 21–26.

Stokes GM, Milner A, Hodges IG & Henry R (1983) Nebulised ipratropium bromide in wheezy infants and young children. *European Journal of Respiratory Research* **64 (supplement 128):** 494–498.

Storr J & Lenney W (1986) Nebulised ipratropium bromide and salbutamol in asthma. *Archives of Disease in Childhood* **61:** 602–603.

Storr J, Barrell E, Barry W & Lenney W (1987) Effect of a single dose of prednisolone in acute childhood asthma. *Lancet* **i:** 879–881.

Strauss RE, Bonggura VR & Valacer DJ (1990) Short course glucocorticosteroids in asthma. *Pediatric Reviews and Communications* **5:** 83–93.

Sur S, Croffy TB, Kephant GM et al (1993) Sudden onset fetal asthma: a distinct entity with genoeosinophils and relatively more neutrophils in the airway submucosa. *American Review of Respiratory Diseases* **148:** 713–719.

Tattersfield A & Barnes P (1992) Beta$_2$-agonists and corticosteroids: new developments and controversies. *American Review of Respiratory Disease* **146:** 1637–1641.

Taylor K & Shaw RJ (1993) The mechanism of action of corticosteroids in asthma. *Respiratory Medicine* **87:** 261–277

Vidgren M (1994) Factors influencing lung deposition of inhaled steroids. *European Respiratory Review* **4:** 68–70.

Warner JO (1992) A follow-up statement from an international paediatric asthma consensus group. *Archives of Disease in Childhood* **67:** 240–248.

Warner JO (1994) The beta-agonist controversy and its relevance to the treatment of children. *European Respiratory Review* **4:** 21–26.

Weinberger M (1993) Theophylline: When should it be used? *Journal of Pediatrics* **122:** 403–404.

Widdicombe J (1993) Neurohumoral mechanisms in obstructive airways disease. In Gross NJ (ed.) *Anticholinergic Therapy in Obstructive Airway Disease,* pp 33–47. London: Franklin Scientific Publications.

Williams TJ & Yarwood H (1990) Effects of glucocorticoid on microvascular permeability. *American Review of Respiratory Disease* **141:** S52–58.

Wrenn K, Sloris CM, Murphy F & Greenberg RS (1991) Aminophylline therapy for acute bronchospastic disease in the emergency room. *Annals of International Medicine* **115:** 241–247.

Yiallouros P & Milner A (1994) Effective pulmonary blood flow in children with acute asthma attack requiring hospitalisation. *Pediatric Pulmonology* **17:** 370–377.

Zainudin BM, Ismail O & Yusoff K (1994) Effect of adding aminophylline infusion to nebulised salbutamol in acute severe asthma. *Thorax* **49:** 267–269.

8

Prophylactic drugs in asthma: their use and abuse

JOHAN C. DE JONGSTE

Drugs for the treatment of asthma are commonly divided into those with direct bronchodilating activity and those which protect against broncho-constricting stimuli without having a direct effect on airway caliber. This last category includes sodium cromoglycate, nedocromil sodium and corticosteroids, drugs which have anti-inflammatory effects but do not relax airway smooth muscle. The term 'prophylactic' to describe agents which lack bronchodilator activity is somewhat confusing, since it pertains to the mode of use rather than to the pharmacological properties of the agent, and bronchodilators give excellent protection too when taken prior to most bronchoconstricting stimuli. In this context we will use the term 'prophylactic' to indicate drugs without direct bronchodilating action that protect against asthmatic airway narrowing to a variety of stimuli.

This chapter reviews the role of prophylactic treatment in asthma with a focus on sodium cromoglycate and topical corticosteroids, because these are first choice for the maintenance treatment of asthma in children and are relatively well documented.

PHARMACOLOGY OF PROPHYLACTIC DRUGS

Cromoglycate

Mechanisms of action

Disodium cromoglycate has been widely used for treating asthma for more than 25 years. The drug was originally thought to act via the inhibition of IgE-mediated release from mast cells, but several other modes of action have been demonstrated as well. Cromoglycate has inhibitory effects on a number of inflammatory cells. It partly inhibits the IgE-mediated release of histamine and other mediators from mast cells in sensitized human lung tissue in concentrations in the micromolar range (Church and Warner, 1985). Interestingly, the release of chemotactic factors, probably from mast cells, is also inhibited by cromoglycate and this may explain part of the broader anti-inflammatory actions that have been observed. In addition, the

Baillière's Clinical Paediatrics—
Vol. 3, No. 2, May 1995
ISBN 0–7020–1986–0

379

activation of eosinophilic and neutrophilic granulocytes, macrophages and platelets may be inhibited by cromoglycate (Kay, 1987; Skedinger et al, 1987; Tunon-de-Lara et al, 1992). The mechanism of these effects has not yet been elucidated, although inhibition of calcium influx at the level of calcium channels has been shown (Spataro and Bosmann, 1976; Kurose, 1981). Cromoglycate has no direct effect on isolated airway smooth muscle contractility. There may be an effect on sensory nerve endings in the airway wall which cause local and central cholinergic reflexes after irritants. Stimulation of these C-fibre endings in the dog airway by capsaicin can be inhibited by cromoglycate in relatively low doses (Richards et al, 1986). However, this has not been confirmed in humans and comparative studies with lignocaine have suggested that cromoglycate may not block irritant receptors in human airways (Persson, 1987). Animal experiments have further suggested that cromoglycate may reduce nerve-mediated mediator release (Biggs and Goel, 1985).

In human skin, cromoglycate attenuates the effect of platelet-activating factor on local oedema formation, and inhibits the response to tachykinins. These findings led to the speculation that cromoglycate may antagonize the action of tachykinins, a mechanism that could also be important in the lungs (Crossman et al, 1994). Cromoglycate could also act on airway vasculature. It prevents histamine-induced plasma leakage from dilated capillaries in the airway mucosa (Persson, 1987), and inhibits hypoxic vasoconstriction (Taylor et al, 1988).

Recent data have demonstrated an inhibiting effect of cromoglycate on IgE production by human B lymphocytes, probably by inhibition of IgE isotype switching (Loh et al, 1994). Although the relevance of this in vitro study to the in vivo situation needs to be confirmed, it adds an interesting mechanism to the many putative actions of cromoglycate that could explain its effect.

To summarize, the anti-asthmatic effect of cromoglycate is based on a well-documented inhibition of mediator and cytokine release from mast cells and other inflammatory cells, and perhaps also on the inhibition of neural reflexes in the airways, either via an effect on nerves or via interaction with neuropeptides. The molecular site of action of cromoglycate remains to be determined.

Direct clinical effects

The protection against allergen-induced bronchoconstriction was the first therapeutic effect of cromoglycate, reported by Altounyan in 1967. Both the immediate bronchoconstriction, and the late allergic reaction can be inhibited effectively by previous administration of cromoglycate.

The effect of cromoglycate persists for several hours after a single dose (Patel and Wall, 1986). For optimal results it should be given every 3–4 hours, and this remains a serious disadvantage for long-term treatment. After inhalation, cromoglycate is partly and rapidly absorbed in the respiratory tract mucosa. Blood levels can be detected and correlated with the clinical effect (Yahav et al, 1988). After inhalation of a single dose of

5–20 mg cromoglycate, immediate dose-dependent protection against a variety of different stimuli can be demonstrated. These stimuli include not only allergens but also exercise (Tullett et al, 1985; Patel and Wall, 1986), hyperventilation of cold dry air (Juniper et al, 1986), inhalation of non-isotonic saline (Kivity et al, 1989; O'Callaghan et al, 1990; Anderson et al, 1994), pollutants such as SO_2 (Koenig et al, 1988), adenosine (Phillips et al, 1989) and metabisulphite (McClellan et al, 1990). Indeed, most of these triggers are believed to act via mast cell activation and/or stimulation of sensory nerve endings. Cromoglycate has no important effect on stimuli that directly activate airway smooth muscle, such as inhaled methacholine or histamine (Lemire et al, 1984; Van Essen-Zandvliet and Kerrebijn, 1990).

Long-term effects

Daily treatment with cromoglycate for several months does not improve airway hyperresponsiveness per se (Van Essen-Zandvliet and Kerrebijn, 1990), although literature data are conflicting and difficult to compare because of different populations and varying treatment durations (Hoag and McFadden, 1991). However, the increase in hyperresponsiveness during the pollen season in atopic asthmatics could be prevented by continuous treatment with cromoglycate for 6 weeks (Löwhagen and Rak, 1985). The transient increase in airway responsiveness that follows the allergic reaction can be reduced by cromoglycate, if treatment is started before the challenge (Mattoli et al, 1987). A major disadvantage of cromoglycate is that the drug has to be taken three or four times daily. It is likely that, in the long term, children will not comply with such a regimen especially when there are few symptoms. This may be one of the reasons why cromoglycate is clinically inferior to inhaled corticosteroids.

Inhaled corticosteriods

Mechanism of action

Corticosteroids are the most effective prophylactic drugs for treating asthma and, since the development of safe and potent preparations for topical use, they have become increasingly important for asthma management. Corticosteroids for topical use in asthma are beclomethasone dipropionate, budesonide and fluticasone propionate. The first two seem clinically equivalent and equipotent. The recently introduced fluticasone seems more potent than beclomethasone or budesonide (Gustafsson et al, 1993). Whether it has a better safety profile with equipotent dosing remains to be established.

Corticosteroids act mainly by interfering with the activities of a variety of inflammatory cells (Barnes and Pedersen, 1993). Corticosteroids act on cytoplasmatic receptors that, after agonist binding, move to the nucleus within minutes, and promote synthesis of a number of specific protein molecules within hours. These include many different proteins that may improve asthma, such as neutral endopeptidase, which inactivates neuro-peptides in the airways, and lipocortin, which inhibits synthesis of arachidonic acid metabolites via an action on phospholipase A_2 in the cell membrane. Steroids thus prevent the secretion of eicosanoid inflammatory mediators and platelet-activating factor. Apart from promoting protein synthesis, steroids also inhibit transcription of genes responsible for pro-inflammatory peptides, such as a number of interleukins, growth factors and tumour necrosis factor, and inducible nitric oxide synthase.

Adherence of inflammatory cells to the endothelium is impaired by steroids because they inhibit the expression of adhesion molecules. Steroids inhibit cytokine and mediator release from eosinophils, neutrophils, macrophages and platelets. Mediator release from mast cells seems resistant to corticosteroids; however, long-term treatment with inhaled steroids reduces the number of mast cells in the airway wall considerably. Microvascular permeability is reduced by corticosteroids, and this may add to their anti-asthmatic activity (Boschetto et al, 1991). This is supported by the uncontrolled observation that the concentration of plasma proteins in lung lavage fluid in asthmatics, which reflects vascular leakage, decreases with steroid treatment (Van de Graaf et al, 1991).

The above mentioned actions of inhaled steroids lead to a pronounced anti-inflammatory effect which has now been documented in adult asthmatics in vivo by means of airway lavage and biopsy studies (Wilson et al, 1994). Numbers of eosinophils, mast cells, lymphocytes and macrophages decrease during steroid treatment for several weeks or months, and their activation state, as measured by the expression of acti-vation markers at the cell surface and production of mediators and cytokines, is reduced (Burke et al, 1992; Djukanović et al, 1992; Jeffery et al, 1992; Duddridge et al, 1993; Wilson et al, 1994). Whether or not inhaled steroids can reverse morphological changes in the airway wall, such as epithelial damage, basement membrane thickening or fibrosis, is question-able. This may require longer treatment periods than have been applied in recent studies (Jeffery et al, 1992; Laitinen et al, 1992).

Steroids have no direct relaxing effect on isolated airway muscle prepa-rations, but can reverse tachyphylaxis to the muscle relaxing effect of β agonists in vitro by increasing the transcription rate of the β_2-receptor gene.

Direct clinical effects

Unlike cromoglycate, inhaled corticosteroids have little if any direct protective effect. Bronchodilatation cannot be shown, the protection against bronchoconstrictor stimuli is negligible (Van Essen-Zandvliet et al, 1993). Inhaled steroids may have other effects, including improvement of mucociliary clearance and increase of β receptor numbers, but their relevance is not well documented in asthmatic humans in vivo. A beneficial effect of inhaled steroids given in the acute phase of viral respiratory tract infections in young children to prevent virus-induced wheeze has been demonstrated, but seems marginal (Connett and Lenney, 1993). There is no reason to believe that inhaled steroids could worsen the course of viral infections (American Academy of Allergy and Immunology, 1993). The use of inhaled steroids in preschool children only during acute asthma attacks does not seem to be very effective, although an improvement in symptom scores was documented in a double-blind study (Wilson and Silverman, 1990). In a recent study, the effects of systemic and inhaled corticosteroids have been compared in 123 children with a mean age of 10 months who presented with acute wheezing. Here, budesonide 0.5 mg every 4 hours led to a significantly more rapid improvement of symptoms than placebo. No significant differences were found between systemic and local steroids which were both more effective than bronchodilator only (Daugbjerg et al, 1993). It is difficult to appreciate these results, because of the small groups and the use of 'soft' endpoints; also, the pathophysiology of the wheezing may vary between subjects within groups.

Long-term effects

After several weeks or months of treatment, inhaled steroids protect against a variety of triggers. There is effective protection against late allergic responses and attenuation of direct allergic reactions (De Baets et al, 1990). The increase in airway responsiveness during allergen exposure can be reduced by inhaled steroids (Boner et al, 1991). Also, exercise-induced asthma is effectively reduced.

Inhaled steroids, given for several months, improve airway responsiveness to various stimuli including pharmacological challenges with histamine or methacholine, adenosine, metabisulphite, exercise, hyperventilation of dry cold air and inhaled aerosols of nonisotonic solutions (Kerrebijn, 1990; Vathenen et al, 1991; O'Connor et al, 1992). Regarding pharmacological challenges, not only the sensitivity to these stimuli, expressed as a provocative dose or concentration, but also the maximal bronchoconstriction after high doses is reduced by inhaled steroids (Bel et al, 1991).

Several studies have been published on the long-term effects of inhaled steroids in young children. At the age of 1–2 years, the diagnosis of asthma is often uncertain, and therefore the term 'recurrent wheezing' is appropriate. Recurrently wheezing infants may well have airway pathology distinct from asthma, such as viral infections and/or relatively narrow or floppy airways, and aspiration of food or gastric content. This is a problem when evaluating specific anti-asthmatic drug effects in this age group. The administration of drugs via the inhaled route is also a problem in infants, and requires either nebulizer systems or valved spacers with a facemask. Such delivery systems will deposit only a small proportion of the drug in the child's lungs (Lødrup Carlsen et al, 1992). Consequently, relatively high doses are needed. Bisgaard et al (1990) found that 3 months of continuous treatment with budesonide 0.8 mg daily via a spacer device reduced exacerbation rate and symptoms in 77 children with a mean age of 2 years, who had recurrent wheezing. Noble et al (1992) confirmed this in a study where 24 children with a mean age of 11 months were given 0.3 mg of budesonide daily via a spacer device. Benefits included fewer symptoms and reduction of comedication. Likewise, Connett et al (1993) found a significant improvement in symptoms and medication-need in a group of 1–3-year-old children who received 0.4–0.8 mg of budesonide daily for 6 months. In preschool children with severe asthma, inhaled steroids reduce the need for systemic steroids (Ilangovan et al, 1993). Small improvements in lung function were shown in a group of asthmatic preschool children who received 0.4 mg of budesonide daily (Greenough et al, 1988). In somewhat older children, benefit was found from 0.3 mg of beclomethasone daily during 6 months (Storr et al, 1986), and from 0.4 mg of budesonide during 6 weeks, with reduction of comedication and improved lung function (Gleeson and Price, 1988).

In summary, a number of relatively small, double-blind controlled studies on the effect of inhaled steroids in preschool children have all shown benefits from several months of daily treatment with conventional doses between 0.3 and 0.8 mg per day. However, most studies have relied on subjective measures of disease severity and not on lung function.

PROPHYLACTIC DRUGS AND ACUTE ASTHMA

Cromoglycate is ineffective when given during acute asthma, although there is a lack of data to support this. If cromoglycate is given after an early asthmatic reaction to allergen, the effects on the late response and the increase in airway responsiveness seem marginal, although a dose-response relationship has not been studied (Cockcroft et al, 1993).

Inhaled corticosteroids have no acute bronchodilator effect, and have only minor direct influence on airway responsiveness (Van Essen-Zandvliet et al, 1993). Therefore, they cannot be recommended for the treatment of severe acute asthma. Small or subjective benefits have been shown from inhaled steroids given for acute episodes of asthma in preschool children, or for virus-induced asthma attacks, where the drug was given after the first symptoms of infection (Wilson and Silverman, 1990; Connett and Lenney, 1993). There is a lack of controlled data on the effect of inhaled steroids in acute severe asthma in older children.

It has been shown that if inhaled steroids are given after an early allergic reaction, they can reduce the late response and the concomitant increase in airway reactivity (Cockcroft et al, 1993). By this mechanism, inhaled steroids may change the course of allergen-induced asthma favourably. Despite theoretical considerations in favour of the use of inhaled steroids in acute asthma, there are few if any clinical studies to confirm the benefits of inhaled steroids for this indication. Conclusive data are needed before the prescription of high-dose inhaled steroids for acute asthma can be recommended.

PROPHYLACTIC DRUGS AND ASTHMA MORBIDITY

Maintenance treatment with cromoglycate reduces asthma symptoms in patients with mild asthma (Hoag and McFadden, 1991). Its effectiveness has also been shown in very young children with recurrent wheezing (Geller-Bernstein and Levin, 1982; Henry et al, 1984; Cogswell and Simpkiss, 1985) and in prematures with neonatal lung damage (Yuksel and Greenough, 1992). Observed benefits in the age group below 2 years were reduced night cough, improved activity, more symptom-free days and less severe asthma as observed by the parents. In schoolchildren with mild asthma, cromoglycate improves symptoms and lung function significantly within a period of 3 months (Furukawa et al, 1984; Shapiro et al, 1988; Selcow et al, 1989). Addition of cromoglycate to a regimen of bronchodilators in children and adults with relatively mild asthma improves symptoms and peak flow values significantly more than placebo in the course of 1 year (Eigen et al, 1987).

Long-term treatment with inhaled corticosteroids reduces asthma morbidity most effectively. Inhaled steroids give a considerable reduction in symptoms and exacerbation rate, and improve baseline lung function, peak flow variability, and airway responsiveness. Inhaled steroids reduce the need for systemic steroids and can often replace maintenance treatment with oral steroids. In a prospective, placebo-controlled study on the effect of inhaled budesonide in 116 children with moderately severe asthma, Van Essen-Zandvliet et al (1992) found that children who received 0.6 mg of budesonide daily had a reduction of symptoms within a few months, together with an improvement of lung function to normal values. The responsiveness of the airways, measured as the provocative dose of methacholine which caused a 20% fall in forced expiratory volume (FEV_1) from baseline, improved consistently but slowly during the whole study period of almost 2 years (Figure 1). The placebo group, with only a β-agonist, showed no improvement and had a high percentage of drop-outs, which could be due to the fact that many of these children had discontinued treatment with inhaled steroids several weeks before entering the study and worsened for that reason. In this study, only a minority of children on

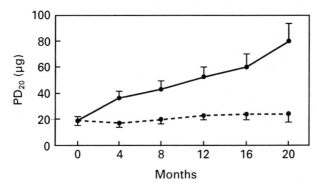

Figure 1. Gradual improvement of airway hyperresponsiveness during long-term treatment with budesonide 0.2 mg three times a day. After 20 months of treatment, the provocative dose of inhaled methacholine that caused a 20% of FEV_1 (PD_{20}, vertical axis) was still rising, and most children were still in the asthmatic range. Reproduced from Van Essen-Zandvliet et al (1992, *American Review of Respiratory Disease* **146:** 547–554) with permission.

inhaled steroids reached a complete remission of their asthma, defined as being symptom-free for 8 months, with no need for rescue medication. In most, airway responsiveness improved and levelled off at values that were still within the asthmatic range (Van Essen-Zandvliet et al, 1994). It seems important to know whether higher doses of inhaled steroids would have done better. The twice-daily dosing regimen makes long-term treatment with inhaled steroids feasible although most children may take only half the prescribed dose even then.

PROPHYLACTIC DRUGS AND ASTHMA MORTALITY

There is relatively strong evidence that systemic corticosteroids, given in the acute phase of a severe asthma attack, are effective and that undertreatment with systemic steroids may result in fatalities. It is much less clear whether or not long-term treatment with inhaled steroids or cromoglycate prevents asthma deaths. There are indications that those who die from asthma or have had life-threatening asthma were grossly undertreated with anti-inflammatory drugs (Molfino and Slutsky, 1994). Careful analysis of fatalities from asthma in the USA and New Zealand revealed undertreatment with specific asthma medications, including prophylactic drugs, as one of the important factors contributing to asthma death in children (Sears et al, 1985; Sly, 1988). Undertreatment was also found in a study on 80 asthma deaths and 154 near-fatal cases from South Australia, where similar levels of undertreatment were found in both groups, and inhaled steroids were only used by 44% of lethal cases and 38% of near-fatal cases (Campbell et al, 1994). Burgess et al (1994) found no difference in the use of inhaled steroids and cromoglycate in a case-control study of 155 patients who had near-fatal asthma attacks. This suggests that patients with severe, life-threatening asthma are undertreated, but perhaps not more than patients with less severe asthma. In a paediatric study, undertreatment with anti-inflammatory drugs was evident in a group of 35 asthma deaths (Fletcher et al, 1990). Thus, several studies support the hypothesis that fatal asthma is related to undertreatment with prophylactic drugs, although it may well be that undertreatment is equally common in non-fatal cases. Specific indications that maintenance treatment with a particular category of prophylactic drugs reduces asthma mortality or near-fatal asthma is lacking. Whether or not undertreatment with inhaled steroids is an independent risk factor or merely reflects a general deficiency in the management, attitude and perception of the disease by either the patient, the parents or the doctor remains unclear.

DO PROPHYLACTIC DRUGS IMPROVE THE LONG-TERM OUTCOME OF ASTHMA?

Controlled long-term studies on the effect of cromoglycate on asthma outcome are lacking. Regarding inhaled steroids, Waalkens et al (1993) have published the results of a prospective, double-blind study on the effect of tapering the dose of inhaled budesonide in asthmatic children who had been treated in a controlled fashion for several years with 0.6 mg of budesonide daily. In this study, a deterioration in lung function, airway responsiveness and return of symptoms was seen in the group in which the dose was reduced over a period of 6 months, whereas the control group remained stable (Figure 2). Although this study was performed in a relatively small

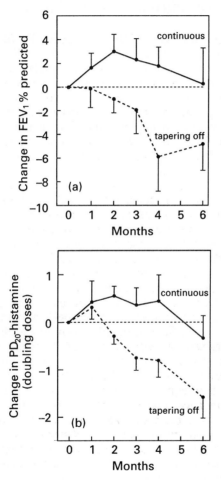

Figure 2. Effects of tapering the dose of inhaled corticosteroids in 28 asthmatic children. After a controlled treatment with inhaled corticosteroids for 28–36 months, the dose of steroids was reduced by 50% every month in 20 children, and a placebo was given for the next 4 months. In the remaining eight, the initial steroid dose of 0.6 mg per day was continued in a randomized, double-blind fashion. The change in baseline FEV_1 (a) and airway responsiveness to histamine, expressed as PD_{20} (b) were compared between those who tapered the dose (– – –) and those who continued (——). The changes in PD_{20} differed significantly between the groups, and were independent of individual levels before tapering. Reproduced from Waalkens et al (1993, *American Review of Respiratory Disease* **148**: 1252–1257) with permission.

group of selected patients, it strongly suggested that even years of daily treatment with inhaled steroids do not alter the long-term outcome of childhood asthma. It may well be, however, that an earlier start of treatment with anti-inflammatory drugs from the outset of the first asthma symptoms has long-term benefits, but in the absence of controlled studies this remains a hypothesis (Selroos, 1991).

SIDE EFFECTS OF PROPHYLACTIC DRUGS

Cromoglycate is remarkably free of side effects. Powder inhalation may cause throat irritation or cough, but is usually well tolerated. Allergic reactions have been reported but seem exceedingly rare. Inhaled cortico-steroids have a very low systemic availability. They are largely inactivated by a first-pass effect in the liver after absorption through the intestinal mucosa, and the main source of systemic activity may therefore be absorption from the lungs. Inhaled steroids do have systemic side effects. These include a suppression of the adrenal cortisol secretion, changes in bone metabolism and growth, and rarely other steroid side effects, perhaps only in persons with abnormal sensitivity (Barnes and Pedersen, 1993). Also, local side effects may be seen, such as throat irritation and hoarseness, thrush, and contact dermatitis. The incidence of oral candidiasis seems very low (Shaw and Edmunds, 1986) and may depend on the delivery system used. Fear that airway mucosal atrophy will result from long-term treatment with inhaled steroids does not seem to be justified. Biopsies of airway mucosa of six adult asthmatic patients who had used inhaled steroids for 10 years had a normal microscopic appearance (Lundgren et al, 1988). Reduction of the circulating numbers of eosinophils and elevated percentages of neu-trophils (both well within the normal range) are seen with conventional doses of inhaled steroids. Inhalation of corticosteroids may produce a small but measurable suppression of the hypothalamo-pituitary-adrenal axis, even at low doses. This has been confirmed in a number of studies, but there are no reports on clinically relevant hypocorticism due to inhaled steroid use. Normal basal and stimulated cortisol secretion was found in 2–7 year-old children who received 0.2 mg of budesonide for 3–5 years (Volovitz et al, 1993). Bisgaard et al (1991) found normal urinary cortisol excretion during treatment with 0.2–0.8 mg of budesonide daily. Dose-dependent suppres-sion of basal cortisol secretion has been documented in children for doses of budesonide and beclomethasone between 0.2 and 1.2 mg per day, in most cases without impairment of the adrenocorticotrophin-stimulated cortisol secretion (Pedersen and Fuglsang, 1987; Bisgaard et al, 1988; Freigang and Ashford, 1990; Phillip et al, 1992; Ninan et al, 1993).

Effects on growth and bone metabolism have been studied extensively and have shown that inhaled steroids may change the blood levels of certain markers of bone metabolism. Osteocalcin and carboxypropeptide of type 1 procollagen were reduced by 0.4–0.8 mg of budesonide daily during several months (Sorva et al. 1992) whereas 0.3–0.8 mg of inhaled beclo-methasone did not affect serum osteocalcin and other markers of bone metabolism in another study in a small group of asthmatic children (König et al, 1993). Bone density as measured by X-ray densitometry showed no effect of conventional doses of beclomethasone (0.2–0.4 mg daily) for at least 6 months compared with matched control asthmatics without steroid treatment (Baraldi et al, 1994). This was, however, a cross-sectional study. Studies on growth in asthmatic children who use inhaled steroids have yielded confusing data. On the one hand, short-term inhibition of the growth of long bones during treatment with conventional doses of budesonide (0.2–0.8 mg daily) or beclomethasone (0.4–0.8 mg daily) has been demonstrated using knemometry, a sensitive technique which measures short-term linear growth of the lower leg (Wolthers and Pedersen, 1991, 1993). With this method, fluticasone 0.2 mg daily seemed to have a smaller inhibiting effect on bone growth than beclomethasone 0.4 mg daily (Wolthers and Pedersen, 1993).

On the other hand, no effects on growth of stature have been observed in several long-term prospective and retrospective studies, even sometimes with high doses for longer periods of time (Nassif et al, 1987; Ninan and Russell, 1992; Van Essen-Zandvliet et al, 1993; Volovitz et al, 1993). In a recent meta-analysis, Allen et al (1994) could find no evidence that either conventional or high (> 0.8 mg daily) doses of inhaled steroids, in particular beclomethasone, reduced final stature.

Another concern has been whether inhaled steroids have an effect on lung and airway growth. This has been evaluated by Merkus (1993), who found normal progression of lung volumes and airway patency after maximal bronchodilatation in asthmatic children with and without inhaled steroids who were followed for several years. These data indicated that normal lung growth can be expected during treatment with inhaled steroids, at least in children of school age. The effect of long-term administration of inhaled steroids in much younger children has not been evaluated. In a short-term study, 0.2 mg of budesonide through a spacer device had no effect on knemometrically-determined lower leg growth in infants, but 0.8 mg caused transient inhibition (Bisgaard, 1993).

Several observations do suggest that individual children may experience growth retardation during treatment with inhaled steroids (Thomas et al, 1994), and this could be due to individual factors that have not been elucidated. In our own experience suggestive growth retardation may be seen in less than 1% of children treated with inhaled steroids. Therefore, it seems important to monitor the growth of each child who receives inhaled steroids carefully, and to adapt the treatment whenever an effect on growth is suspected. It should be borne in mind however, that asthma itself affects growth and delays puberty (Hindmarsh et al, 1993), and that the small risk of side effects from inhaled steroids must be balanced against their powerful anti-asthmatic effect.

Other systemic effects of topical corticosteroids have been reported. These include increase of serum lipids, and insulin/glucose ratios during glucose tolerance tests (Turpeinen et al, 1991), hypertension, ocular cataract and skin bruising (Barnes and Pedersen, 1993). These are, however, extremely rare.

Although the systemic effects of inhaled steroids may be clinically irrelevant or rare, it seems prudent to administer the lowest dose that controls symptoms in such a way that systemic absorption is kept minimal. For this purpose, the use of spacer devices (Brown et al, 1990; Farrer et al, 1990) and mouth rinsing after inhalation can be advised.

THE AIM OF PROPHYLACTIC DRUG TREATMENT IN CHILDHOOD ASTHMA

All prophylactic agents discussed in this chapter have anti-inflammatory actions; nevertheless they are different. Cromoglycate can reduce the acute effect of asthma triggers, and perhaps the transient increase in airway inflammation that follows these triggers, but its effects on chronic airway inflammation and baseline airway responsiveness have not been demonstrated convincingly. In contrast, inhaled corticosteroids can improve chronic airway inflammation in asthma irrespective of recent triggers, and improve airway hyperresponsiveness gradually and consistently. The term 'anti-inflammatory' is rather fuzzy and can mean different things.

The rationale of using steroids or cromoglycate in moderate to severe asthma, but not in mild asthma, is based on the recognition that chronic airway inflammation is the underlying pathophysiological mechanism, and that frequent symptoms are associated with more severe inflammation than mild, infrequent symptoms. Motives for starting maintenance treatment with prophylactic drugs are: firstly, that they provide an important reduction in symptoms and in the need for other medication; and, secondly, that they interfere with the underlying pathophysiological process at a more basal level than bronchodilators, which has led to the speculation that they may improve the long-term outcome. For the purpose of effective reduction of symptoms, prophylactic treatment can be reserved for patients with frequent symptoms who often take daily medications anyhow. For this category, evidence has accumulated to show the superiority of maintenance treatment with inhaled steroids above bronchodilators only (Van Essen-Zandvliet et al, 1992). However, inflammation is probably also present in the airways of patients with mild asthma, and it can be reasoned that by giving anti-inflammatory drugs to children with mild asthma the consequences of ongoing inflammation on the structure of the airways, which may be important in the persistence and severity of symptoms in the long run, could be prevented. Theoretically, there is every reason to consider early and continuing use of effective and safe anti-inflammatory medication in properly selected young asthmatics, aiming at a beneficial effect on the long-term prognosis. However, in view of the lack of evidence that any treatment improves the long-term outcome of childhood asthma, it is at present premature to advise such a strategy other than in the form of a controlled trial. Selection of patients should include demonstration of chronic inflammation as the cause of symptoms, and this is at present not feasible without invasive techniques, such as bronchoscopy and broncho-alveolar lavage. Clearly, we need well designed clinical studies to resolve the issue whether or not early anti-inflammatory treatment improves the prognosis of childhood asthma. For that purpose the development of ethically acceptable, noninvasive techniques to monitor asthmatic airway inflammation in children has a high priority.

In summary, both bronchodilator and anti-inflammatory treatment should be regarded as symptomatic as long as it has not been shown that they improve the long-term prognosis of asthma. Empirically, a much better result can be obtained in moderate to severe asthma with daily anti-inflammatory drugs than with regular use of bronchodilators only and this is the main rationale for their use.

WHICH DRUG FOR WHICH CHILD? EXISTENT GUIDELINES AND ALTERNATIVES

Recent international guidelines for the treatment of asthma in children advise maintenance treatment with cromoglycate in case of frequent symptoms for which bronchodilators are needed several days per week, and switching to inhaled steroids when at least 6 weeks of cromoglycate are unsuccesful. Steroids are primarily indicated when the asthma is severe. The severity of asthma is estimated from bronchodilator use, symptoms and peak flow variations (Warner, 1992). There is some ambiguity in the guidelines especially because the effect of treatment is included in the judgement of severity. The need for bronchodilators varies widely between individuals and may not reflect correctly asthma severity; peak flow variation patterns are often not stable and sometimes difficult to obtain in young children. Also, it is unclear how to decide after 6 weeks of cromoglycate if the effect was good enough, especially because many parents and patients will greatly appreciate a slight improvement, while perhaps more could have been gained initially with stronger medication. Finally, this 'step-up' guideline has the disadvantage that increasing the medication if the effect is not satisfactory may take a lot of time and demotivate the patient. An alternative 'step-down' approach has been advocated by different experts. It may yield better results much quicker and motivate the patient to continue his treatment, that should be tapered to the lowest level that provides adequate control. In this approach, the initial treatment is inhaled steroids in conventional or even high doses, followed by tapering as soon as the desired improvement has been reached, and eventually replacing the steroids by cromoglycate (Figure 3).

Obviously, it is difficult to make strict recommendations on treatment schedules on the basis of present insufficient knowledge, which is that prophylactic treatment reduces symptoms and improves lung function while it is used. As yet there seems no reason to prefer steroids above cromoglycate in children in whom cromoglycate is very effective; treatment with inhaled steroids should always be monitored carefully to detect possible rare side effects.

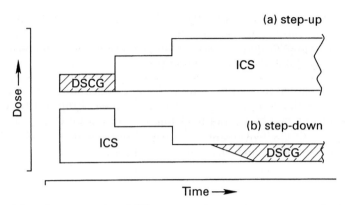

Figure 3. Schematic representation of different approaches to asthma management in children. (a) Step-up approach as advised in various consensus articles. (b) Step-down approach, which may result in more rapid improvement and better compliance. Which of the two is best remains to be shown. DSCG = disodium cromoglycate; ICS = inhaled corticosteroid.

USE AND ABUSE OF PROPHYLACTIC DRUGS IN CHILDHOOD ASTHMA

Preferably, drugs should be prescribed only for indications where their effects have been proven. If we recognize that cromoglycate is mainly active as a short-acting prophylactic that protects against a variety of asthma triggers, it may rationally be given daily to children who encounter these triggers so often, e.g. on most days, that daily protection is justified and acceptable. The prophylactic use of cromoglycate prior to infrequent challenges on an as-needed base seems unpractical: Inhaled β-agonists will do better, and make treatment simpler because no second drug is needed.

It could be argued that if a child is so hyperresponsive that it has symptoms on most days and after many triggers, the use of cromoglycate as a short-term prophylactic is inferior to the use of steroids. The strong emphasis on inhaled steroids, that comes from adult chest medicine where the pathophysiology of asthma and the effects of steroids have been studied extensively, has the risk of overuse and abuse in paediatrics, where it is often unclear whether or not respiratory symptoms are due to asthmatic airway inflammation or to other transient, often benign pathology that does not require anti-inflammatory treatment. Recently, concern has risen about the possible overuse of inhaled steroids for nonspecific airway symptoms in young children. It was proposed to limit their use to those children in whom asthma substantially interferes with a normal lifestyle or in whom there is persisting airways obstruction (Phelan, 1994). The data on acute application of inhaled steroids in preschool children with respiratory symptoms as discussed above are suggestive of a small beneficial effect, but rely on subjective endpoints and short-term observations. The effect on outcome after several months or years is not clear. Hence, there is no reason yet for a liberal use of inhaled corticosteroids in young children with nonspecific respiratory symptoms like cough or wheeze.

WHEN SHOULD PROPHYLACTIC AGENTS BE CEASED?

As soon as the asthma has been in remission for several months, which means that there have been no symptoms and a normal lung function without the need for bronchodilators, the question arises if treatment can safely be discontinued. The maximal improvement from inhaled steroids is reached at different time points for different outcome measures. The improvement in symptoms and lung function characteristically is reached long before the improvement in airway responsiveness (Van Essen-Zandvliet et al, 1994), and this indicates that a lack of symptoms does not necessarily mean that the underlying pathology in the airways has disappeared. It is, however, unusual to do serial measurements of airway responsiveness or repeated bronchoscopies to follow the results of treatment, and not all experts agree whether hyperresponsiveness is the thing to treat. As an increased responsiveness not only reflects inflammation of the airway, but also structural changes of airways and parenchyma that may not respond to steroids, the concept that responsiveness should be treated with anti-inflammatory drugs is probably invalid.

Tapering of steroid treatment in asthmatic children who are in remission while taking steroids has a high probability of relapse of symptoms, airway hyperresponsiveness and airway obstruction (Waalkens et al, 1993). It appeared that worsening may occur within a period of several months after each stepwise reduction of steroid dose.

If the asthma has been in remission for some time, e.g. 6 months, an attempt can be made to reduce the steroid dose by, for example, one quarter. After each dose step, the frequency and severity of asthma symptoms should be observed carefully and, if possible, peak flow recordings should be obtained after a period of 2–3 months before a next step is undertaken. It is important to take the effect of external factors into account as well. Reducing prophylactic treatment just before a season with a great probability of worsening, such as the pollen season or the cold season, is often disappointing. It is not clear whether or not it is useful to measure airway responsiveness each time before the dose of corticosteroids is reduced; relapses may occur even when hyperresponsiveness has disappeared.

SUMMARY

The availability of effective and safe prophylactic drugs for the treatment of asthma has made it possible to achieve control of symptoms and normalization of lung function in most children with moderate to severe asthma. Fortunately, this treatment is very safe and, although systemic effects of inhaled corticosteroids are detectable, clinically relevant side effects are rare. The choice between cromoglycate and steroids is largely determined by the severity of the symptoms. Cromoglycate is still considered first choice for those children with moderate asthma in whom adequate symptom control can be reached with the drug. This is mainly because of the small risks of steroid side effects, that specifically worries paediatricians who favour the use of a nonsteroidal anti-inflammatory treatment, especially in young children. When steroids are used, it is important to monitor for possible systemic effects, especially growth retardation which may be seen occasionally. The presently recommended 'step-up' treatment schedule needs to be reconsidered and the merits of alternative 'step-down' schedules should be investigated. There is a lack of data on possible beneficial effects of prophylactic treatment on the long-term outcome of childhood asthma. Theoretical considerations lead to the early and long-term use of anti-inflammatory drugs, but the available data are not convincing and long-term prospective studies are needed before firm recommendations can be made. In the meanwhile, anti-inflammatory treatment should not be withheld as long as the asthma is problematic and interferes with normal activities.

REFERENCES

Allen DB, Mullen ML & Mullen B (1994) A meta-analysis of the effect of oral and inhaled corticosteroids on growth. *The Journal of Allergy and Clinical Immunology* **93:** 967–976.

American Academy of Allergy and Immunology (1993) Position statement: Inhaled corticosteroids and severe viral infections. *The Journal of Allergy and Clinical Immunology* **92:** 223–228.

Anderson SD, Du Toit JI, Rodwell LT & Jenkins CR (1994) Acute effect of sodium cromoglycate on airway narrowing induced by 4.5 percent saline aerosol. *Chest* **105:** 673–680.

Baraldi E, Bollini MC, De Marchi A & Zacchello F (1994) Effect of beclomethasone dipropionate on bone mineral content assessed by X-ray densitometry in asthmatic children: a longitudinal evaluation. *European Respiratory Journal* **7:** 710–714.

Barnes PJ & Pedersen S (1993) Efficacy and safety of inhaled corticosteroids in asthma. *American Review of Respiratory Disease* **148:** S1–S26.

Bel EH, Timmers MC, Zwinderman AH et al (1991) The effect of inhaled corticosteroids on the maximal degree of airway narrowing to methacholine in asthmatic subjects. *American Review of Respiratory Disease* **143:** 109–113.

Biggs DF & Goel V (1985) Mechanisms of action of sodium-cromoglycate. *Canadian Journal of Physiology and Pharmacology* **63:** 760–765.

Bisgaard H (1993) Systemic activity of inhaled topical steroid in toddlers studies by knemometry. *Acta Paediatrica* **82:** 1066–1071.

Bisgaard H, Pedersen S, Damkjaer Nielsen M & Østerballe O (1991) Adrenal function in asthmatic children treated with inhaled budesonide. *Acta Paediatrica Scandinavia* **80:** 213–217.

Bisgaard H, Damkjaer Nielsen M, Andersen B et al (1988) Adrenal function in children with bronchial asthma treated with beclomethasone dipropionate or budesonide. *Journal of Allergy and Clinical Immunology* **81:** 1088–1095.

Bisgaard H, Munch SL, Nielsen JP et al (1990) Inhaled budesonide for treatment of recurrent wheezing in early childhood. *The Lancet* **336:** 649–651.

Boner AL, Piacentini GL, Bonizzato C et al (1991) Effect of inhaled beclomethasone dipropionate on bronchial hyperreactivity in asthmatic children during maximal allergen exposure. *Pediatric Pulmonology* **10:** 2–5.

Boschetto P, Rogers DF, Fabbri LM & Barnes PJ (1991) Corticosteroid inhibition of airway microvascular leakage. *American Review of Respiratory Disease* **143:** 605–609.

Brown PH, Blundell G, Greening AP & Crompton GK (1990) Do large volume spacer devices reduce the systemic effects of high dose inhaled corticosteroids? *Thorax* **45:** 736–739.

Burgess C, Pearce N, Thiruchelvam R et al (1994) Prescribed drug therapy and near-fatal asthma attacks. *European Respiratory Journal* **7:** 498–503.

Burke C, Power CK, Norris A et al (1992) Lung function and immunopathological changes after inhaled corticosteroid therapy in asthma. *European Respiratory Journal* **5:** 73–79.

Campbell DA, Mclennan G, Coates JR et al (1994) A comparison of asthma deaths and near-fatal asthma attacks in South Australia. *European Respiratory Journal* **7:** 490–497.

Church MK & Warner JO (1985) Sodium cromoglycate and related drugs. *Clinical Allergy* **15:** 311–320.

Cockcroft DW, McParland CP, O'Byrne PM et al (1993) Beclomethasone given after the early asthmatic response inhibits the late response and the increased methacholine responsiveness and cromolyn does not. *The Journal of Allergy and Clinical Immunology* **91:** 1163–1168.

Cogswell JJ & Simpkiss MJ (1985) Nebulised sodium cromoglycate in recurrently wheezy preschool children. *Archives of Disease in Childhood* **60:** 736–738.

Connett G & Lenney W (1993) Prevention of viral induced asthma attacks using inhaled budesonide. *Archives of Disease in Childhood* **68:** 85–87.

Connett GJ, Warde C, Wooler E & Lenney W (1993) Use of budesonide in severe asthmatics aged 1–3 years. *Archives of Disease in Childhood* **69:** 351–355.

Crossman DC, Dashwood MR, Taylor GW et al (1993) Sodium cromoglycate: evidence of tachykinin antagonist activity in human skin. *The Journal of Applied Physiology* **75:** 167–172.

Daugbjerg P, Brenøe E, Forchhammer H et al (1993) A comparison between nebulized terbutaline, nebulized corticosteroid and systemic corticosteroid for acute wheezing in children up to 18 months of age. *Acta Paediatrica* **82:** 547–551.

De Baets FM, Goeteyn M & Kerrebijn KF (1990) The effect of two months of treatment with inhaled budesonide on bronchial responsiveness to histamine and house-dust mite antigen in asthmatic children. *American Review of Respiratory Disease* **142:** 581–586.

Djukanović R, Wilson JW, Britten KM et al (1992) Effect of an inhaled corticosteroid on airway inflammation and symptoms in asthma. *American Review of Respiratory Disease* **145:** 669–674.

Duddridge M, Ward C, Hendrick DJ & Walters EH (1993) Changes in bronchoalveolar lavage inflammatory cells in asthmatic patients treated with high dose inhaled beclomethasone dipropionate. *European Respiratory Journal* **6:** 489–497.

Eigen H, Reid JJ, Dahl R et al (1987) Evaluation of the addition of cromolyn sodium to bronchodilator maintenance therapy in the long-term management of asthma. *The Journal of Allergy and Clinical Immunology* **80:** 612–621.

Farrer M, Francis AJ & Pearce SJ (1990) Morning serum cortisol concentrations after 2 mg inhaled beclomethasone dipropionate in normal subjects: effect of a 750 ml spacing device. *Thorax* **45:** 740–742.

Fletcher HJ, Ibrahim SA & Speight N (1990) Survey of asthma deaths in the Northern region, 1970–85. *Archives of Disease in Childhood* **65:** 163–167.

Freigang B & Ashford DR (1990) Adrenal cortical function after long-term beclomethasone aerosol therapy in early childhood. *Annals of Allergy* **64:** 342–344.

Furukawa CT, Shapiro GG, Bierman W et al (1984) A double-blind study comparing the effectiveness of cromolyn sodium and sustained-release theophylline in childhood asthma. *Pediatrics* **74:** 453–459.

Geller-Bernstein C & Levin S (1982) Nebulized sodium cromoglycate in the treatment of wheezy bronchitis in infants and young children. *Respiration* **43:** 294–298.

Gleeson JGA & Price JF (1988) Controlled trial of budesonide given by the Nebuhaler in preschool children with asthma. *British Medical Journal* **297:** 163–166.

Greenough A, Pool J, Gleeson JGA & Price JF (1988) Effect of budesonide on pulmonary hyperinflation in young asthmatic children. *Thorax* **43:** 937–938.

Gustafsson P, Tsanakas J, Gold M et al (1993) Comparison of the efficacy and safety of inhaled fluticasone propionate 200 µg/day with inhaled beclomethasone dipropionate 400 µg/day in mild and moderate asthma. *Archives of Disease in Childhood* **69:** 206–211.

Henry RL, Hiller EJ, Milner AD et al (1984) Nebulised ipratropium and sodium cromoglycate in the first two years of life. *Archives of Disease in Childhood* **59:** 54–57.

Hindmarsh PC, Crowley S & Brook CGD (1993) Effects of asthma and asthma treatment on children's growth. *European Respiratory Review* **3:** 313–316.

Hoag JE & McFadden ER (1991) Long-term effect of sodium cromolyn on nonspecific bronchial hyperresponsiveness: a review. *Annals of Allergy* **66:** 53–63.

Ilangovan P, Pedersen S, Godfrey S et al (1993) treatment of severe steroid dependent preschool asthma with nebulised budesonide suspension. *Archives of Disease in Childhood* **68:** 356–359.

Jeffery PK, Godfrey RW, Ädelroth E et al (1992) Effects of treatment on airway inflammation and thickening of basement membrane reticular collagen in asthma. *American Review of Respiratory Disease* **145:** 890–899.

Juniper EF, Latimer KM, Morris MM et al (1986) Airway responses to hyperventilation of cold dry air: Duration of protection by cromolyn sodium. *The Journal of Allergy and Clinical Immunology* **78**: 387–391.

Kay AB (1987) The mode of action of anti-inflammatory drugs. *Clinical Allergy* **17**: 153–164.

Kerrebijn KF (1990) Use of topical corticosteroids in the treatment of childhood asthma. *American Review of Respiratory Disease* **141**: S77–S81.

Kivity S, Ganem R, Greif J & Topilsky M (1989) The combined effect of nifedipine and sodium cromoglycate on the airway response to inhaled hypertonic saline in patients with bronchial asthma. *European Respiratory Journal* **2**: 513–516.

Koenig JQ, Marshall SG, Van Belle G et al (1988) Therapeutic range cromolyn dose-response inhibition and complete obliteration of SO_2-induced bronchoconstriction in atopic adolescents. *The Journal of Allergy and Clinical Immunology* **81**: 897–901.

König P, Hillman L, Cervantes C et al (1993) Bone metabolism in children with asthma treated with inhaled beclomethasone dipropionate. *Journal of Pediatrics* **122**: 219–226.

Kurose M (1981) Inhibition of anaphylactic histamine release from heterologously sensitized mast cells: differential effects of drugs which interfere with calcium influx. *Acta Medica Okayama* **35**: 307–317.

Laitinen LA, Laitinen A & Haahtela T (1992) A comparative study of the effects of an inhaled corticosteroid, budesonide, and B_2-agonist, terbutaline, on airway inflammation in newly diagnosed asthma: A randomized, double-blind, parallel-group controlled trial. *The Journal of Allergy and Clinical Immunology* **90**: 32–42.

Lødrup Carlsen KC, Nikander K & Carlsen K-H (1992) How much nebulised budesonide reaches infants and toddlers? *Archives of Disease in Childhood* **67**: 1077–1079.

Lemire I, Cartier A, Malo J-L et al (1984) Effect of sodium cromoglycate on histamine inhalation tests. *The Journal of Allergy and Clinical Immunology* **73**: 234–239.

Loh RKS, Jabara HH & Geha RS (1994) Disodium cromoglycate inhibits $S\mu{\to}S^-$ deletional switch recombination and IgE synthesis in human B cells. *Journal of Experimental Medicine* **180**: 663–671.

Löwhagen O & Rak S (1985) Modification of bronchial hyperreactivity after treatment with sodium cromoglycate during pollen season. *The Journal of Allergy and Clinical Immunology* **75**: 460–467.

Lundgren R, Söderberg M, Hörstedt P & Stenling R (1988) Morphological studies of bronchial mucosal biopsies from asthmatics before and after ten years of treatment with inhaled steroids. *European Respiratory Journal* **1**: 883–889.

Mattoli S, Foresi A, Corbo GM et al (1987) Effects of two doses of cromolyn on allergen-induced late asthmatic response and increased responsiveness. *The Journal of Allergy and Clinical Immunology* **79**: 747–754.

McClellan MD, Wanger JS & Cherniack RM (1990) Attenuation of the metabisulfite-induced bronchoconstrictive response by pretreatment with cromolyn. *Chest* **97**: 826–830.

Merkus PJFM (1993) Growth of lungs and airways in asthma. PhD Thesis, University of Rotterdam.

Molfino NA & Slutsky AS (1994) Near-fatal asthma. *European Respiratory Journal* **7**: 981–990.

Nassif E, Weinberger M, Sherman B & Brown K (1987) Extrapulmonary effects of maintenance corticosteroid therapy with alternate-day prednisone and inhaled beclomethasone in children with chronic asthma. *The Journal of Allergy and Clinical Immunology* **80**: 518–529.

Ninan TK & Russell G (1992) Asthma, inhaled corticosteroid treatment, and growth. *Archives of Disease in Childhood* **67**: 703–705.

Ninan TK, Weid IW, Carter PE et al (1993) Effects of high doses of inhaled corticosteroids on adrenal function in children with severe persistent asthma. *Thorax* **48**: 599–602.

Noble V, Ruggins NR, Everard ML & Milner AD (1992) Inhaled budesonide for chronic wheezing under 18 months of age. *Archives of Disease in Childhood* **67**: 285–288.

O'Callaghan C, Milner AD & Swarbrick A (1990) Nebulised sodium cromoglycate in infancy: airway protection after deterioration. *Archives of Disease in Childhood* **65**: 404–406.

O'Connor BJ, Ridge SM, Barnes PJ & Fuller RW (1992) Greater effect of inhaled budesonide on adenosine 5'-monophosphate-induced than on sodium-metabisulfite-induced bronchoconstriction in asthma. *American Review of Respiratory Disease* **146**: 560–564.

Patel KR & Wall RT (1986) Dose-duration effect of sodium cromoglycate aerosol in exercise-induced asthma. *European Journal of Respiratory Diseases* **69**: 256–260.

Pedersen S & Fuglsang G (1988) Urine cortisol excretion in children treated with high doses of inhaled corticosteroids: a comparison of budesonide and beclomethasone. *European Respiratory Journal* **1**: 433–435.

Persson C (1987) Cromoglicate, plasma exudation and asthma. *Trends in Pharmacological Sciences* **8:** 202–203.

Phelan PD (1994) Asthma in children: epidemiology. *British Medical Journal* **308:** 1584–1585.

Phillip M, Aviram M, Leiberman E et al (1992) Integrated plasma cortisol concentration in children with asthma receiving long-term inhaled corticosteroids. *Pediatric Pulmonology* **12:** 84–89.

Phillips GD, Scott VL, Richards R & Holgate ST (1989) Effect of nedocromil sodium and sodium cromoglycate against bronchoconstriction induced by inhaled adenosine 5'-monophosphate. *European Respiratory Journal* **2:** 210–217.

Richards IM, Dixon M, Jackson DM & Vendy K (1986) Alternative modes of action of sodium cromoglycate. *Agents and Actions* **18:** 294–300.

Sears MR, Rea HH, Beaglehole R et al (1985) Asthma mortality in New Zealand: a two-year national study. *New Zealand Medical Journal* **98:** 271–275.

Selcow JE, Mendelson LM & Rosen JP (1989) Clinical benefits of cromolyn sodium aerosol (MDI) in the treatment of asthma in children. *Annals of Allergy* **62:** 195–199.

Selroos O (1991) The effects of inhaled corticosteroids on the natural history of obstructive lung disease. *European Respiratory Review* **1:** 354–365.

Shapiro GG, Furukawa CT, Pierson WE et al (1988) Double-blind evaluation of nebulized cromolyn, terbutaline, and the combination for childhood asthma. *The Journal of Allergy and Clinical Immunology* **81:** 449–454.

Shaw NJ & Edmunds AT (1986) Inhaled beclomethasone and oral candidiasis. *Archives of Disease in Childhood* **61:** 788–790.

Skedinger MC, Augustine NH, Morris EZ et al (1987) Effect of disodium cromoglycate on neutrophil movement and intracellular calcium mobilization. *The Journal of Allergy and Clinical Immunology* **80:** 573–577.

Sly RM (1988) Mortality from asthma in children 1979–1984. *Annals of Allergy* **60:** 433–443.

Sorva R, Turpeinen M, Juntunen-Backman K et al (1992) Effects of inhaled budesonide on serum markers of bone metabolism in children with asthma. *The Journal of Allergy and Clinical Immunology* **90:** 808–815.

Spataro AC & Bosmann HB (1976) Mechanism of action of disodium cromoglycate—mast cell calcium ion influx after a histamine-releasing stimulus. *Biochemical Pharmacology* **25:** 505–510.

Storr J, Lenney CA & Lenney W (1986) Nebulised beclomethasone dipropionate in preschool asthma. *Archives of Disease in Childhood* **61:** 270–273.

Taylor BJ, Fewell JE & Kearns GL (1988) Pulmonary vascular response to aerosolized cromolyn sodium and repeated epochs of isocapneic alveolar hypoxia in lambs. *Pediatric Research* **23:** 513–518.

Thomas BC, Stanhope R & Grant DB (1994) Impaired growth in children with asthma during treatment with conventional doses of inhaled corticosteroids. *Acta Paediatrica* **83:** 196–199.

Tullett WM, Tan KM, Wall RT & Patel KR (1985) Dose-response effect of sodium cromoglycate pressurised aerosol in exercise induced asthma. *Thorax* **40:** 41–44.

Tunon-de-Lara JM, Rio P, Marthan R et al (1992) The effect of sodium cromoglycate on platelets: An in vivo and in vitro approach. *The Journal of Allergy and Clinical Immunology* **89:** 994–1000.

Turpeinen M, Sorva R & Juntunen-Backman K (1991) Changes in carbohydrate and lipid metabolism in children with asthma inhaling budesonide. *The Journal of Allergy and Clinical Immunology* **88:** 384–389.

Van de Graaf EA, Out TA, Roos CM & Jansen HM (1991) Respiratory membrane permeability and bronchial hyperreactivity in patients with stable asthma. *American Review of Respiratory Disease* **143:** 362–368.

Van Essen-Zandvliet EEM & Kerrebijn KF (1990) The effect of antiasthma drugs on bronchial hyper-responsiveness. *Immunology and Allergy Clinics of North America* **10:** 483–501.

Van Essen-Zandvliet EEM, Hughes MD, Waalkens HJ et al (1992) Effects of 22 months of treatment with inhaled corticosteroids and/or beta-2-agonists on lung function, airway responsiveness, and symptoms in children with asthma. *American Review of Respiratory Disease* **146:** 547–554.

Van Essen-Zandvliet EEM, Hop WCJ, De Jong H et al (1993) Minor acute effect of an inhaled corticosteroid (budesonide) on bronchial hyperresponsiveness to methacholine in children with asthma. *European Respiratory Journal* **6:** 383–386.

Van Essen-Zandvliet EEM, Hughes MD, Waalkens HJ et al (1994) Remission of childhood asthma after long-term treatment with an inhaled corticosteroid (budesonide): Can it be achieved? *European Respiratory Journal* **7:** 63–68.

Vathenen AS, Knox AJ, Wisniewski A & Tattersfield AE (1991) Effect of inhaled budesonide on bronchial reactivity to histamine, exercise, and eucapnic dry air hyperventilation in patients with asthma. *Thorax* **46:** 811–816.

Volovitz B, Amir J, Malik H et al (1993) Growth and pituitary—adrenal function in children with severe asthma treated with inhaled budesonide. *New England Journal of Medicine* **329:** 1703–1708.

Waalkens HJ, Van Essen-Zandvliet EEM, Hughes MD et al (1993) Cessation of long-term treatment with inhaled corticosteroid (budesonide) in children with asthma results in deterioration. *American Review of Respiratory Disease* **148:** 1252–1257.

Warner JO (1992) Asthma: a follow-up statement from an international pediatric asthma consensus group. *Archives of Disease in Childhood* **67:** 240–248.

Wilson JW, Djukanović R, Howarth PH & Holgate ST (1994) Inhaled beclomethasone dipropionate downregulates airway lymphocyte activation in atopic asthma. *American Journal of Critical Care Medicine* **149:** 86–90.

Wilson NM & Silverman M (1990) Treatment of acute, episodic asthma in preschool children using intermittent high dose inhaled steroids at home. *Archives of Disease in Childhood* **65:** 407–410.

Wolthers OD & Pedersen S (1991) Growth of asthmatic children during treatment with budesonide: a double blind trial. *British Medical Journal* **303:** 163–165.

Wolthers OD & Pedersen S (1993) Short term growth during treatment with inhaled fluticasone propionate and beclomethasone diproprionate. *Archives of Disease in Childhood* **68:** 673–676.

Yahav Y, Dany S, Katznelson D & Farfei Z (1988) Sodium cromoglycate in asthma: correlation between response and serum concentrations. *Archives of Disease in Childhood* **63:** 592–597.

Yuksel B & Greenough A (1992) Inhaled sodium cromoglycate for preterm children with respiratory symptoms at follow-up. *Respiratory Medicine* **86:** 131–134.

9

Allergy in childhood asthma

CHRISTIAN H. L. RIEGER

Allergy is an untoward physiological reaction mediated through immunologic mechanisms (Farr and Spector, 1975)

Until the beginning of the 20th century asthma was interpreted as a disease of 'autonomic imbalance'. Trigger factors, among others, were considered to be exercise, changing weather or 'coldness and humidity of the spirit'. After demonstration of the allergic shock in the guinea-pig the pathophysiological concept of asthma changed drastically, so much that in 1947 Cooke stated 'if asthma is an allergy and only an allergy, as I believe, the factors such as worry, excitement, psychic trauma, psychasthenia, vasomotor instability, autonomic imbalance, exertion, endocrine disorder, fatigue, exposure to cold and dampness, fumes or gases are not of basic importance.'

The present concept of the role of allergy in asthma is more complex. It is true that the available evidence suggests the presence of allergy, or more specifically, an atopic disposition, in over 90% of children with asthma and that in these patients specific IgE is detected against one or even a variety of airborne allergens, food or other substances. Nevertheless, specific IgE against a given allergen may not be related to the patient's disease. If it does cause an asthmatic reaction, it may do so consistently or only at times when additional factors concur. Specific IgE irrelevant to the patient's bronchial mucosa may cause an inflammation to the nose or sinuses thus indirectly affecting his asthma. Specific IgE, for example against food, may trigger an asthmatic reaction early in life and become irrelevant later. The opposite is true for allergens causing rhinitis if the patient later develops asthma.

Specific IgE, the hallmark of atopy, may then be regarded as a necessary prerequisite for the development of childhood asthma. It is insufficient, however, in most if not all patients to cause disease without additional coexisting factors and it may change its significance to a patient or to single organs over time. Understanding the characteristics of allergens and their interplay with other factors in the generation of the bronchial reaction is one of the keys to understanding the pathophysiology of asthma.

Baillière's Clinical Paediatrics—
Vol. 3, No. 2, May 1995
ISBN 0–7020–1986–0

399

GENETICS

A genetic disposition is a prerequisite for the development of manifest allergic disease (Table 1). It is clear that asthma 'runs in families' but the type of heredity and the specific defect have not been clarified yet. It is obvious to think that such defect should either generate bronchial hyper-reactivity unrelated to atopy or specifically predispose to allergic sensitization at the level of the bronchus-associated immune system thus creating bronchial reactivity as a phenomenon secondary to allergic inflammation.

The first mentioned concept is supported by the observation that in infants with a family history of asthma, bronchial hyperresponsiveness can be demonstrated by an increased histamine response shortly after birth. Also, bronchial hyperreactivity can be seen in nonallergic and in symptom-free individuals and appears to follow a genetic pattern (Landau, 1992).

The second concept would represent hyperreactivity secondary to allergic inflammation. As mucosal inflammation varies over time this type of bronchial hyperreactivity, although characteristic of any population of asthmatics, does not correlate with disease severity in an individual patient. Moreover, it may not even be consistently demonstrable in a given patient. In a recent study of asthmatic children, bronchial hyperreactivity was seen in only two out of three of the group at a given time (Pattemore et al, 1990).

The two concepts are clearly not mutually exclusive, but seem to predominate independently at least to some degree. Allergy appears to be the more important factor in the generation of childhood asthma since it can cause bronchial hyperreactivty. However it does depend on the persistence of nonspecific hyperreactivity to become symptomatic whereas bronchial hyperreactivity without allergy is found even in nonasthmatics.

Research on molecular genetics in asthma and atopy has identified two chromosomes as possible candidates for 'atopy', or even 'asthma-genes'. One analysis of 43 families suggested an autosomal dominant mode of inheritance for atopy. The putative gene was linked to the long arm of chromosome 11 (Cookson and Hopkin, 1988). This finding has not been confirmed by other laboratories.

More recently, an investigation of 11 Amish families with IgE to inhalant allergens was able to link five markers in chromosome 5q 31.1 to a gene

Table 1. Development of manifest allergy.

Genetic disposition	Allergen	Manifest Allergy
Probability		
no atopic parent 10–15%		Living conditions
one atopic parent 20–35%		Smoking parents
two atopic parents 55–80%		Bottle-feeding
		Outdoor pollution
		Infections
		Unknown environmental conditions

controlling total serum IgE concentration. Interestingly, these studies found evidence that the gene identified controls interleukin 4 production thus regulating IgE in a nonantigen specific fashion (Marsh et al, 1994).

In the clinical study by Kjellmann (1977) on allergies in 1325 7-year-old Swedish children, disease developed in 19.8% with a single parent history, in 42.9% with a double family history, and in 72.2% of children with parents having the same atopic manifestation.

SENSITIZATION AND ASTHMA

The determinants for bronchial sensitization and the initiation of the asthma process are not completely understood. Antigen exposure very early in life, i.e. during the first 6 months, seems important, since a higher incidence of pollen allergy is found in infants born in spring whereas a higher incidence of mite allergy occurs among those born in the autumn (Björkstén and Kjellmann, 1990). Also, the incidence of mite asthma during later childhood can clearly be related to the level of allergen exposure during the first year of life (Sporik et al, 1990). Exposure to pets during the first 6 months of life is followed by a higher incidence of sensitization (Munir, 1994). The importance of early life for the development of allergy is also shown by population studies which demonstrated that migration after the first year of life resulted in an asthma prevalence characteristic of the community from which the child came, whereas migration before birth resulted in the prevalence of asthma characteristic of the community where the child eventually grew up (Hurry et al, 1988).

It is of interest that in experimental animals a critical period exists early in life during which tolerance to allergens develops under physiological conditions (Holt et al, 1990). In guinea pigs transient asthma to inhaled ovalbumin can be induced by adding ovalbumin to the animals' food for a period of 3 to 4 weeks (Riedel et al, 1989). A transient increase to IgE anti-ovalbumin is also seen in normal infants aged 6–12 months (Hattevig et al, 1993). It is conceivable that triggering of the asthma–allergy process is somehow connected to the physiological process of tolerance-induction. Factors inducing or facilitating the process of sensitization, besides atopy, include maternal smoking, air pollution, viral infections, bottle feeding and prematurity.

There is good evidence that the increasing incidence of asthma in the Western world parallels the increase of allergies in general. A striking example of this is the doubling of the asthma incidence among Tokelauans following their migration from Tokelau to New Zealand (White et al, 1980). As the genetic make-up of humans has not changed during recent decades, environmental factors must account for the phenomenon in some way. Air pollutants such as SO_2, O_3 and NO_2, NO_3 (nitrous oxide) have been incriminated and can clearly facilitate allergic sensitization under experimental conditions. Also, allergies are more frequent in children living in polluted areas compared to control populations within the same country (Andrae et al, 1988).

On the other hand, a comparison of asthma frequency in East and West Germany following reunification found a much higher incidence of asthma and specific IgE in West Germany in spite of greater concentrations of air pollutants in the eastern part of the country (von Mutius et al, 1994). Accordingly, other factors, e.g. parasite infestation, must additionally be assumed to influence immune-regulation with regard to allergic sensitization.

The intimate link between asthma and allergy can be documented in many ways.

(i)   More than 80% of asthmatic children possess specific IgE against one or more allergens.

(ii)   A total of 28–61% of asthmatic children have allergic rhinitis and 50% have atopic dermatitis (Smith, 1993).

(iii) A family history of atopy is present in the majority of asthmatic children.

(iv)   Even in the absence of specific IgE, bronchial provocation with allergens can produce a reaction in some patients.

(v)   Asthma was exceedingly rare before 'westernization' and the advent of allergies in developing countries. The sudden appearance of asthma along with mite allergy in New Guinea is a striking example of such an association (Dowse et al, 1985).

'INTRINSIC ASTHMA'

There is the occasional patient with cough and recurrent wheeze who has no evidence of atopic disposition, no historical link between exposure to airborne allergens, symptoms and negative provocation tests. Sweat test and DNA analysis have ruled out cystic fibrosis with more than 95% probability, ciliary function is normal, immunodeficiency is excluded as best as possible, structural anomalies such as tumours or fistulas are ruled out, the parents do not smoke and the patient was a healthy baby born at term. The term 'intrinsic asthma' usually applied to such children, is unfortunate since it does not constitute a diagnosis but merely excludes IgE as a pathogenic factor.

These patients show severe chronic inflammation on bronchial biopsy which is indistinguishable from allergic asthma. The pathogenesis of this type of asthma remains unclear in most cases. Pseudo-allergy, i.e. non IgE-mediated triggering of mast cells, basophils and other inflammatory cells must be considered, however. One agent responsible for such events can be aspirin which causes a known syndrome of asthma and nasal polyps. These patients may also react to indomethacin, to other nonsteroidal anti-inflammatory agents and to tartrazin yellow, a dye used as a food colouring agent in many foods and drugs (Smith and Slavin, 1976; Fuglsang et al, 1994). It should also be remembered that inflammatory cells such as eosinophils or neutrophils can be recruited by T-cells in response to allergens without the help of IgE and mast cells.

At present, the nature of most non IgE-mediated asthma is unclear. It exists in a small minority of asthmatic children and may well be closely related to atopic asthma.

ALLERGENS

Airborne substances capable of sensitizing humans and eliciting an allergic inflammation on re-exposure are usually categorized as mite-, pollen-, animal- and mold-allergens. Other allergens, e.g. cockroaches and other insects, increasingly add to the list (Lierl et al, 1994). The pathogenic significance of these allergens for paediatric asthma is quite variable.

Specific IgE-antibodies against mites, *Dermatophagoides pteronyssimus* and *Dermatophagoides farinae*, are present in a large proportion of asthmatic children depending on their place of residence. Sporik et al, for example, found a 94% incidence of mite sensitization among 11-year-old English children with asthma, whereas in northern Sweden only 2% of asthmatics are sensitized (Sporik et al, 1990; Wickmann et al, 1993). Worldwide, the major antigens of mites constitute by far the most important allergen for the asthmatic child. Major mite allergens include Der pI, Der pII, Der fI and Der fII. Der pI is an excretory product of the mite. The Der pII and Der fII cDNAs have been cloned and sequenced. They share 88% homolgy.

Mites thrive best under warm and humid conditions; they cannot exist in high altidudes. Highest concentrations of mites are found in matresses containing organic material, in woollen blankets, feather pillows, toy pets, carpets and upholstery.

The effect of mite allergens on mite-sensitive asthma can be demonstrated in various ways. If such a patient moves to a high altitude, his asthma will disappear both clinically and by lung function measurement within 1–2 months. Similarly, decreased bronchial reactivity follows reduction of domestic exposure to mites (Ehnert et al, 1992). Conversely, a single inhalation of the allergen under laboratory conditions can cause a dual asthmatic reaction which may leave the patient with bronchial hyperreactivity for as long as 6 weeks. Chronic exposure to mite antigen is the most likely explanation for the background inflammation seen in many asthmatics which seems to set the stage for clinical reactions to other allergens and to nonspecific triggers which would otherwise go unrecognized. For example, exercise and humidity were unknown to cause bronchial obstruction in New Guinea before the advent of mite-induced asthma and are now recognized as frequent trigger mechanisms.

The degree of mite sensitivity obviously varies from patient to patient. It seems, at least to some degree, to be determined by the level of exposure during the first 6 months of life (Luczynska et al, 1990; Sporik et al, 1990). Even in the same patient the tolerance or reactivity to mites varies over time and may be influenced by upper respiratory infections, intensity of previous exposure, coexistence of other allergies and by nonspecific irritants such as smoking or air polluton.

Although there is no doubt as to the role of mites in the pathogenesis of bronchial asthma it may be difficult to prove their significance in the individual patient, e.g. when immunotherapy is considered. Bronchial provocation is unreliable while the patient is on medication and is dangerous when he is symptomatic. Immediate responses can occur in patients with specific IgE even if they have no asthma. Finally, both particle size and quantities of allergen used in bronchial provocation are different from natural exposure.

Other insect allergens which cause and sustain asthmatic symptoms come from cockroaches and possibly various other insects against which specific IgE has been demonstrated. Cockroaches seem to be of particular relevance in American homes. Removal is very difficult due to the high resistance of cockroaches to chemicals.

The role of pollen-allergens for childhood asthma is more complex to understand than that of other allergens. Most pollen grains will reach the lung only by mouth-breathing since they are cleared by the nose due to their size. This may be one reason why their significance is greater in allergic rhinitis than in asthma. They also cause recurrent bronchial obstruction but in a pattern which is not only seasonal but also dependent on other factors such as respiratory infections (Busse, 1990), concurrent exposure to mites and other perennial allergens, and possibly to nonspecific irritants. Which type of pollen is of particular importance to groups of patients depends on their residential area. While in Europe grass pollen, birch, alder, willow and hazelnut cause most reactions, short ragweed is by far the most important allergen in the midwest of the United States and cedar pollen in Japan.

Several of the major allergens of these pollen are meanwhile cloned, e.g. Lol pI, Lol pII, and Lol pIII, the major allergens of rye grass, *Lolium pratense*; or Amb aI and Amb aII, the two major allergens of short ragweed. The only tree pollen studied in detail is the birch pollen. One major allergen, Bet VI and one minor allergen, Bet VII, have been cloned (Markert, 1992).

Pollen extracts show quite variable concentrations of single allergens. This may be due to yearly differences in climatic conditions but possibly also to environmental factors such as air pollution. In fact, major allergens of birch were shown to be more frequently expressed by trees in polluted areas (Breiteneder and Scheiner, 1991). Along with the known variation in pollen counts due to weather changes these qualitative changes of pollens explain at least part of the extremely variable allergen load the individual patient meets during the season. In addition, coexisting allergic rhinits leading to mouth-breathing, increased bronchial reactivity resulting from exposure to mites, pets and other allergens, air pollution or viral infections will increase the asthma provoking effect of pollen. Taken together, the number of factors determining the bronchial reaction to pollen allergens (Table 2) is so remarkable that the individual disease course cannot be predicted from one season to the next.

Animals as a source of allergens are third in importance to the asthmatic child but particularly difficult to deal with. If a gerbil or guinea-pig is the culprit, an acceptable solution is not so difficult to reach. Cats and dogs, on

Table 2. Factors determining the reaction to pollen.

Preceding viral upper respiratory infections
Background inflammation due to other allergen
Previous exposure to the same allergen (time of season)
Allergen content of pollen
Individual pattern of reactivity
Pollen count
Air pollution
Coexisting allergic rhinitis
Time spent outside
Medication

the other hand, are so frequent in Western civilization that allergy control is never complete even after permanent removal of the animal from the child's home.

The most significant animal allergen comes from the cat. Termed Feld DI, it is found in saliva, fur, skin and urine (Bartholomé et al, 1985; Luczynska et al, 1990). Once the saliva is dry the albumin obviously is distributed into the cat's environment. Dust probes, accordingly, will contain cat allergen not only in homes but also in schools and other places where children meet.

Dog allergens may not be as aggressive but due the frequency of dogs in modern homes and due to the intimate contact between children and most dogs their dander is another rich source of allergens (Spitzauer, 1994).

When taking an allergy history, it is important to inquire about birds as parents may not mention them in response to a more general question. Birds like parrots or parakeets have a particularly effective way of rendering their dust particles airborne and definitely constitute a major source of allergenic exposure.

While the number of possible allergenic animals is endless, horse allergy should be mentioned specifically. Horse dander can cause a remarkable sensitivity. A horse even if kept kilometers away on a farm may be sufficient to maintain allergic symptoms in a child even if contact is restricted to a sibling or classmate.

Practising allergists are often full of stories of how a patient may react to his own pet but not to others and therefore will escape detection by allergy testing. This is possible but infrequent.

A Swedish study investigating the sensitivity of prick testing for dog allergy found a sensitivity of 67–88% for various dog breed-allergen preparations. Significant differences between the skin response to different dog breed skin extract preparations, indicating dog breed-specific allergens, was obtained in 15% of their patients. There was no significant correlation between skin prick test results and symptoms relating to a specific breed (Lindgren et al, 1988).

Molds are another important source of allergen in childhood asthma. Frequency of sensitization depends mainly on living conditions, although high concentrations of molds occur outside in temperate climate zones, particulary in August and September. In humid climates and under poor housing conditions molds often cause a polysensitization and persistent asthmatic symptoms. As molds represent a major source of food for house-dust mites, their presence is of special importance to the asthmatic child.

To suspect mold sensitivity by taking an allergy history may be quite difficult as mold growth can occur in innocent-appearing places, e.g. behind cupboards, under carpets, in walls or even in a child's inhalation device. Most allergists test for the five major types; *Penicillium notatum, Cladosporium herbarum, Aspergillus fumigatus, Mucor racemosus* and *Alternaria tenuis*. In a child with persistent symptoms and suspected mold allergy it should be remembered, however, that there are many more types of molds.

Food and food additives will cause bronchial obstruction during anaphylactic reactions. To what extent they can trigger normal asthmatic attacks or sustain allergic inflammation of the bronchi is not very well documented but appears to affect under 10% of children with proven allergy to food or food additives.

A list of allergens which can cause asthma is given in Table 3.

Table 3. Allergens in asthma

Indoor allergens	
Acarids	Mites, spiders
Insects	Cockroaches, moths, flies
Domestic animals	Cats, dogs, birds
Rodents	Rabbits, gerbils, guinea-pigs, mice, rats, hamsters
Fungi	*Alternaria, Cladosporium, Penicillium, Mucor, Aspergillus*
Outdoor allergens	
Animals	Horses, cows
Insects	Bees, wasps, midges
Pollen	Weeds, trees, grasses, flowers
Fungi	*Alternaria, Cladosporium, Penicillium, Mucor, Aspergillus*

DIAGNOSIS OF SENSITIZATION

In the diagnosis of allergy, chest physicians, paediatricians, allergists and pharmaceutical companies have invested much effort to develop tests to define more clearly the immunological basis of the patients' hypersensitivity. The best known and most widely practised approach are skin tests for the diagnosis of type one reactivity. This method is cheap and reliable if done properly. At present, most centres practise percutaneous testing, the so-called prick test. For this procedure, the patient must not be taking antihistamines for at least 4 days prior to testing and the procedure must be carried out in such a way that the epidermis is perforated but does not bleed. Negative and positive controls (0.9% NaCl and histamine) are to be applied with each testing. Skin reactions must be read after 20 minutes. Reactions are considered positive when they reach at least 3 mm in diameter, in poor responders at least the size of the histamine wheel.

For the serological determination, radioimmunoassays and enzyme linked immunoassays have been developed. They are expensive and not necessary for routine testing of atopic patients. They are well suited, however, for control of skin tests, for patients with atopic eczema and diffuse skin involvement, for small children, for patients with unusually strong dermographism, or if a patient is to be evaluated who has received antihistamines within the last 4 days.

As positive reactions indicate the presence of specific IgE but not its clinical significance, efforts have been undertaken to find appropriate tests for this purpose. Inhalation provocation with allergens, for example, has been widely done using mite, pollens and other allergens. These tests have produced interesting and helpful information on the bronchial response to allergens but for a number of reasons are less than ideal for clinical routine. The main reason for the limited significance of these tests is the fact that they can only be done when the patient is well. At this time, however, he will be much less likely to react than following a viral infection, with impaired nose-breathing or when there is background inflammation following inhalation of another allergen.

Basophil-release assays, the determination of eosinophil cationic protein (Jutunen-Backman et al, 1993), and endoscopic intrabronchial challenge (in adults) were further attempts to find tests with higher clinical significance. All of these attempts have suffered from the fact that the allergen to be tested is rarely the single aetiologic factor for the patient's asthma.

From a practical standpoint inhalation challenges or comparable tests are not as necessary as they may seem. If a child with positive skin reactions to mite or cat has asthma, allergy control measures are required, whether there is a positive inhalation challenge or not. The significance of seasonal allergens is easily documented by history or clinical observation unless the patient is polysensitized. In this case hyposensitization, the only consequence for which a positive challenge would be desirable, cannot be done anyway.

IMMUNOTHERAPY

Since the beginning of the century the application of allergens in increasing amounts has been used to treat allergic disease. Extracts from pollens, animal dander, house dust and other material has been injected and fed to children and adults with the aim of reducing the need for medication or control symptoms completely. Immunotherapy for bee and wasp sting allergy has long been generally accepted as the treatment of choice for systemic reactions. The injection of allergen extracts for treatment of respiratory allergies has, on the other hand, been a subject of controversy for decades. This is understandable since the extracts used were crude and not standardized until recently, and were often applied injudiciously. Attempts to correlate effects on the immune system with the treatment and with clinical success were difficult to obtain and were limited to the demonstration of an increase of IgG-antibodies, which were called 'blocking antibodies'.

At present, a more positive and optimistic view is developing again

among immunologists. Careful investigation of patients under immunotherapy has shown a number of consistent changes which include a
decrease of total and specific IgE, an increase of IgA in nasal secretions, an
effect on antigen-induced eosinophil activation, i.e. the late phase reaction,
a decrease of IgE-receptor-bearing cells and a decrease of platelet activating factor in serum (van Bever et al 1988; Hsieh and Ng, 1993; Bousquet
and Michel, 1994; Makoto and Masanori, 1994).

Secrist et al (1993) have demonstrated that the quantity of interleukin 4
produced by allergen specific memory CD4 positive T-cells from allergic
patients could be considerably reduced by in vivo treatment with allergen
immunotherapy. This effect was more pronounced the longer treatment was
applied. Interleukin 4 is the cytokine responsible for stimulation of IgE-
producing B-cells and at present considered the key substance for the
development of atopy (Secrist et al, 1993).

Clinically there is good evidence that immunotherapy when carried out
correctly is successful in reducing symptoms of seasonal allergic rhinitis
and conjunctivitis caused by pollen in at least 80% of affected patients. The
success of immunotherapy for asthma is more difficult to show as asthmatic
symptoms even in pollen-allergic individuals depend on many other factors
besides pollen count and the individual degree of sensitization. Viral
infections, concurrent mite sensitivity, nonspecific triggers and other
factors determine the clinical course at least as much. Nevertheless, a
number of studies have shown an improvement of symptom scores or an
increase of the provocative dose causing a 20% decrease of forced
expiratory volume in one second (FEV_1) to allergen (Bousquet, 1994).

As perennial allergens, in particular mite allergens, are more significant
in provoking and sustaining childhood asthma, a possible effect of
immunotherapy on mite allergy has been investigated repeatedly. Using
standardized extracts of *Dermatophagoides pteronyssinus* or *Dermatophagoides farinae* a number of studies have been successful in reducing
symptoms although to varying degrees (Warner et al, 1978). There have
been very few successful studies on immunotherapy to cats and dogs.
Obviously, in this type of allergy, removal of the animal is more appropriate.
In particular, as cat allergen is an almost ubiquitous allergen, environmental
control in a highly sensitized child may not be easy, and in an exceptional
patient immunotherapy might be considered (Van Metre et al, 1988).

Successful trials have been carried out using standardized extracts of
Cladosporium herbarum and *Alternaria tenuis* (Malling et al, 1986; Horst
et al, 1990). As molds frequently cause polysensitization and allergy,
control measures are always mandatory and these studies would appear to
be more of theoretical interest.

At present immunotherapy can be regarded as a form of therapy which
affects the immune regulation on the T-cell level and which may be
successful in reducing asthmatic symptoms in individual and well selected
patients. Its role in the overall treatment of childhood asthma is nevertheless small for a number of reasons. The ideal candidates for immunotherapy, children who are allergic to one or two kinds of pollen but not to
any other substance, are rare and their asthma is usually easy to control.

Furthermore, patients who are allergic to perennial allergens will not benefit from injections without environmental control. Following removal of pets and appropriate measures against mites their disease is either no longer a problem or the patient has an unusual degree of sensitization in which case he often has too many types of sensitization for immunotherapy.

It is still unknown which epitopes induce IgE and which are important for the induction of tolerance. In spite of the definite improvement in the quality of extracts, better charactarization of allergens and individualized treatment with defined epitopes remains the goal for the future. It seems very likely that atopy is a disease of the T-cell and that consequently the regulation of T-cell responses has the best prospect for successful treatment of allergic reactions.

PREVENTION

With an incidence of childhood asthma in the range of 10–20% of all school children, preventive measures have become a major issue. Some aspects, for example outdoor pollution, have to be solved on a political level. Others, such as prematurity or respiratory syncytial virus infection are important areas of medical research. Indoor environment and infant nutrition, however, are at least as important and patient education in this area should accordingly have a good chance to reduce allergic respiratory disease.

Allergy prevention begins with the question of who is at risk. A number of immunological markers have been described which characterize infants at risk of atopy, above all an elevated cord blood IgE. Neither this nor any other parameter is nearly as sensitive as the family history to identify infants at risk and to motivate parents. With an almost 10% chance of developing atopy, even in the absence of a positive family history, some recommendations should be given to all couples.

The most important factor, according to our present understanding, is the reduction of mite allergen. A well ventilated and dry home will stay free of molds, the main source of nutrition for mites and a source of allergen itself. A bed with a mattress cover of polyurethane and artificial fibre pillows will keep the bed mite-free. Toy pets must be washable and a carpet, if present, should be kept clean with a vacuum cleaner containing a high efficiency particulate filter. Intense exposure to the sun will also kill mites living in a carpet (Tovey and Woolcock, 1994). It is often amazing, how readily parents will provide all this for their new baby and then take the infant into their own mite-infested bed each night. Consequently, the parents' bedroom and the siblings' bed must be included in the preventive measures. In some countries chemical treatment of carpets with acaricides is recommended. This is unnecessary with the above described measures and has been shown to fail (Huss et al, 1994).

Pets are the second most important indoor allergen. Exposure to a cat or dog during the first 6 months of life carries an increased risk of becoming sensitized. Giving away an animal may sometimes be difficult. In addition, it takes months after removal of the animals before allergens are effectively cleared from the home. This type of counselling should accordingly be done in early pregnancy.

Smoking is a known risk factor. In spite of all pessimism most pregnant women will reduce or quit smoking because they understand the possible harm they do to their child. Why should it not be possible then to extend this awareness to the period after birth? Breast-feeding has become more popular again in industrialized countries. The duration of breast-feeding, however, is insufficient and motivation suffers from the impression that hydrolysed cow milk formulas are as good for allergy prevention. This may be true for infantile eczema but has not been shown for respiratory allergies. Breastmilk protects against respiratory infections, e.g. by stimulating active SIgA-production of the infant, and has many other effects which artificial formulas do not provide. Recommending 6 months of exclusive breast-feeding to an infant at risk of allergy should therefore be part of any comprehensive prevention program.

Allergy is the single most important factor in childhood asthma. Its control through education of families as well as political measures is one of the most important challenges of our time.

SUMMARY

Allergy is present in over 90% of infants and children with bronchial asthma and constitutes the single most important aetiologic factor of this disease. Consequently, the incidence of asthma has increased worldwide in parallel to the rising incidence of allergies. The genetic basis of asthma has not been elucidated yet but recent work points to a gene locus on chromosome 5 which may upregulate the production of interleukin 4 leading to increased concentrations of IgE. The most important allergen in temperate and warm climate zones is the house dust mite which is primarily responsible for the mucosal background inflammation in asthmatics leading to bronchial hyperreactivity and perennial symptoms. Other non-seasonal significant allergens are domestic animals, cockroaches and molds. Reduction or even control of asthmatic symptoms through environmental measures against mites are effective. Hyposensitization currently plays a minor role in the treatment of asthma but has the prospect of becoming an effective tool in the future. The development of asthma in infants and children can probably be controlled to a considerable degree by preventive measures such as encasing of mattresses, avoiding feather pillows and woollen blankets, control of smoking and by ventilating homes more effectively.

REFERENCES

Andrae S, Axelson O, Björkstén B et al (1988) Symptoms of bronchial hyperreactivity and asthma in relation to environmental factors. *Archives of Disease in Childhood* **63**: 473–478.
Bartholomé K, Kissler W, Bear H et al (1988) Where does cat allergen come from? *Journal of Allergy and Clinical Immunology* **76**: 503–506.

van Bever HP, Bosmans J, De Clerck LS & Stevens WS (1988) Modification of the late asthmatic reaction by hyposensitization in asthmatic children allergic to house dust mite (*Dermatophagoides pteronyssinus*) or grass pollen. *Allergy* **43**: 378–386.

Björkstén B & Kjellmann N–I (1990) Perinatal factors influencing the development of allergy. *Clinical and Experimental Allergy* **20**: 3–8.

Bousquet J & Michel FB (1994) Specific immunotherapy in asthma: Is it effective? *The Journal of Allergy and Clinical Immunology* **94**: 1–11.

Breiteneder H & Scheiner O (1991) Umwelt und Allergenexpression. *Internist* **32**: 602–605.

Busse WW (1990) Respiratory infections: their role in airway responsiveness and the pathogenesis of asthma. *The Journal of Allergy and Clinical Immunology* **85**: 671–683.

Cooke RC (1947) *Allergy in theory and Practice*. Philadelphia: Saunders.

Cookson WOCM & Hopkin JM (1988) Dominant inheritance of atopic IgE-responsiveness. *Lancet* **1**: 86–88.

Dowse GK, Turner KJ, Stewart GA et al (1985) The association between Dermatophagoides mites and the increasing prevalence of asthma in village communities within the Papua New Guinea highlands. *The Journal of Allergy and Clinical Immunology* **76**: 75–83.

Ehnert B, Lau–Schadendorf S, Weber A et al (1992) Reducing domestic exposure to dust mite allergen reduces bronchial hyperreactivity in sensitive children with asthma. *The Journal of Allergy and Clinical Immunology* **90**: 135–138.

Farr RS. Spector SL (1975) *What is Asthma? The Asthmatic Patient in Trouble*. Greenwich: CPC Communications Inc.

Fuglsang G, Madsen G, Halken S et al (1994) Adverse reactions to food additives in children with atopic symptoms. *Allergy* **49**: 31–37.

Hattevig G, Kjellman B & Björkstén B (1993) Appearance of IgE antibodies to ingested and inhaled allergens during the first 12 years of life in atopic and non-atopic children. *Pediatric Allergy and Immunology* **4**: 182–186.

Holt PG, McMenamin C & Nelson D (1990) Primary sensitization to inhalent allergens during infancy. *Pediatric Allergy and Immunology* **1**: 3–13.

Horst M, Hejjaoui A, Horst V et al (1990) Double-blind, placebo-controlled rush immunotherapy with a standardized Alternaria extract. *The Journal of Allergy and Clinical Immunology* **85**: 460–472.

Hsieh KH & Ng CK (1993) Increased plasma platelet-activating factor in children with acute asthmatic attacks and decreased in vivo and in vitro production of platelet-activating factor after immunotherapy. *The Journal of Allergy and Clinical Immunology*, **91**: 650–657.

Hurry VM, Peat JK & Woolcock AJ (1988) Prevalence of respiratory symptoms, bronchial hyper-responsiveness and atopy in schoolchildren living in the Villawood area of Sydney. *Australian and Newzealand Journal of Medicine* **18**: 745–752

Huss RW, Huss K, Squire EN & Carpenter GB (1994) Mite allergen control with acaricide fails. *The Journal of Allergy and Clinical Immunology* **1**: 27–32.

Juntunen–Backman K, Järvinen P & Sorva R (1993) Serum eosinophil cationic protein during treatment of asthma. *The Journal of Allergy and Clinical Immunology* **92**: 34–39.

Kjellmann NIM (1977) Atopic disease in seven-year old children. *Acta Paediatrica Scandinavica* **66**: 465–471.

Landau LI (1992) Development of respiratory symptoms and bronchial hyperresponsiveness in infancy. *Pediatric Allergy and Immunology* **3**: 61–65.

Lierl MB, Riodan MM & Fischer TJ (1994) Prevalence of insect allergenspecific IgE in allergic asthmatic children in Cincinnati, Ohio. *Annals of Allergy* **72**: 45–50.

Lindgren S, Berlin L, Drebor S et al (1988) Breedspecific dog-dandruff allergens. *The Journal of Allergy and Clinical Immunology* **82**: 196–204.

Luczynska CM, Li Y & Chapmann MD (1990) Airborne concentrations and particle size distribution of allergen derived from domestic cats (*Felis domesticus*). *American Review of Respiratory Disease* **141**: 361–367.

Makoto N & Masanori S (1994) Specific immunotherapy reduces the antigen-dependent production of eosinophil chemotactic activity from mononuclear cells in patients with atopic asthma. *The Journal of Allergy and Clinical Immunology* **8**: 160.

Malling HJ, Dreborg S & Weeke B (1986) Diagnosis and immunotherapy of mould allergy. V. Clinical efficacy and side effects of immunotherapy with *Cladosporium herbarum*. *Allergy* **41**: 507–519.

Markert ML (1992) Molecular biology and allergy: current status and future prospects. *Pediatric Allergy and Immunology* **92**: 49–60.

Marsh DG, Neely JD, Breazeale DR et al (1994) Linkage analysis of IL4 and other chromosome 5q31.1 markers and total serum immunoglobulin E concentrations. *Science* **264**: 1152–1156.

Munir AKM (1994) Exposure to indoor allergens and relation to sensitization and asthma in children. Thesis, Linköping.

Van Metre TE, Marsh DG & Adkinson NF (1988) Immunotherapy for cat asthma. *The Journal of Allergy and Clinical Immunology* **82**: 1055–1068.

von Mutius E, Martinez FD, Fritzsch C et al (1994) Prevalence of asthma and atopy in two areas of West and East Germany. *American Journal of Respiratory and Critical Care Medicine* **149**: 358–364.

Pattemore PK, Asher MI & Harrison AC (1990) The interrelationship among bronchial hyper-responsiveness, the diagnosis of asthma and asthma symptoms. *American Review of Respiratory Disease* **142**: 549–554.

Riedel F, Kanter N, Schauer U et al (1989) Bronchial sensitization in guinea pigs following ingestion of ovalbumin. *International Archives of Allergy and Applied Immunology* **90**: 395–399.

Secrist H, Chelen CJ, Wen Y et al (1993) Allergen immunotherapy decreases interleukin-4 production in CD4⁺ T-cells from allergic individuals. *Journal of Experimental Medicine* **178**: 2123–2130.

Smith L (1993) Childhood asthma: Diagnosis and treatment. *Current Problems in Pediatrics* **23**: 271–305.

Smith L & Slavin RG (1976) Drugs containing tartrazin dye. *The Journal of Allergy and Clinical Immunology*: **58**: 456–470.

Spitzauer, S (1994) Molecular characterization of dog albumin as a cross-reactive allergen. *The Journal of Allergy and Clinical Immunology* **3**: 614–628.

Sporik R, Holgate ST & Cogswell JJ (1990) Exposure to house dust mite allergen (der p I) and the development of asthma in childhood. A prospective study. *New England Journal of Medicine* **23**: 502–507.

Tovey ER & Woolcock AJ (1994) Direct exposure of carpets to sunlight can kill all mites. *The Journal of Allergy and Clinical Immunology* **93**: 1072–1075.

Warner JO, Price JF, Soothill JF et al (1978) Controlled trial of hyposensitization of *Dermatophagoides pteronyssinus* in children with asthma. Lancet **ii**: 912–916.

White DA, Eyles EF, Tonkin SL & O'Donnell TV (1980) Asthma prevalence in Tokelauan children in two environments. *Clinical Allergy* **120**: 71–75.

Wickmann M, Nordvall SL, Pershagen G et al (1993) Sensitization to domestic mites in a cold temperate region. *American Review of Respiratory Disease* **148**; 58–62.

10

The adolescent with asthma

GLENN BOWES

There is no evidence to suggest that the pathophysiological mechanisms of the disease asthma are any different in young people than in adults. However, it is clear that the unique setting of adolescence mandates a different approach to the clinical care of adolescents with asthma. Implicit to this discussion is that the key principles of treatment of the disease asthma, detailed elsewhere, are incorporated in the asthma management plan. Knowledge of and familiarity with state of the art, scientifically-informed treatment of the airway inflammatory disease we recognize as asthma, is absolutely necessary for the good clinical care of adolescents with asthma—but of itself, not sufficient. Understanding and knowing how to implement developmentally appropriate strategies of clinical care complete the range of skills required for a clinician to manage adolescents with asthma effectively.

DEFINITION OF ADOLESCENCE

Adolescence is the transitional stage of development that occurs between the relative dependency of childhood and the relative independency of adulthood. The term *adolescent* refers to an individual between the age of 10 and 19 years. As a consequence of the increasing recognition that the period of adolescence has become relatively prolonged in contemporary society, the term *young person* is increasingly being used to refer to those individuals between the age of 10 and 24 years.

It is important for clinicians to recognize and monitor the dynamic developmental changes occurring in their adolescent patients and appropriately adjust both the style and mode of their clinical care.

GOALS OF THERAPY: DEVELOPMENTAL AND DISEASE

Clear goals of therapy need to be established for adolescents with asthma. Individualized treatment goals need to be negotiated and set in the context of the young person's life.

Adolescent development involves multiple dimensions including

Baillière's Clinical Paediatrics—
Vol. 3, No. 2, May 1995
ISBN 0–7020–1986–0

413

physiological growth, puberty, cognitive maturation and psychosocial development. Developmental outcomes related to these processes need to be seen as important health outcomes alongside those outcomes that are desirable as a consequence of the treatment of asthma. The psychosocial maturation of adolescents may be seen as a series of developmental tasks and it is natural that these tasks are a dominant focus in the thinking of young people.

Developmental and disease outcomes are listed in Figure 1 to indicate both the parallel focus of clinical management that is required and the potential for significant interactions to occur between the disease and the young person. It is common to see a conflict of priorities occur between the asthma treatment outcomes that are the aim of the clinician and the developmental outcomes that are the goal of the young person. Resolving this conflict by open discussion and the negotiation of mutually agreed upon goals is an important task for clinicians.

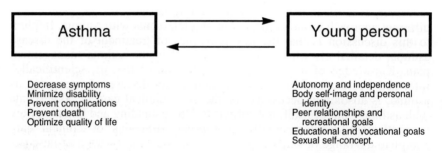

Figure 1. Goals of therapy in adolescents with asthma. Both developmental and disease outcomes need consideration. Arrows indicate significant interactions between asthma and the individual.

YOUNG PEOPLE AND FAMILY

The care of young people with asthma necessitates a consideration of family issues. Asthma has the potential to affect family dynamics significantly and these may be aggravated by the emergence of normal adolescent behaviour.

Achieving the most appropriate balance between continuing parental involvement and progressive adolescent independence is a challenging task for the clinician. Whilst a gradual handing over of responsibility for asthma management from parent to young person is desirable, it is inappropriate for parents to completely withdraw their involvement. More commonly, concerned parents behave in a way that adolescents perceive as overprotective and it is the role of the clinician to act as an advocate for the young person by negotiating with parents to stand back a little from their intensive involvement in the care of asthma in their teenager.

As a young person progresses through adolescence with the continuing presence of asthma, it becomes apparent to parents that their child will not 'grow out' of asthma. A re-emergence of parental guilt may occur as parents more clearly see that their children will live into adult life with an ongoing illness.

COMPLIANCE

Compliance with treatment regimens is an issue in the management of all people with asthma. Although there is little data to support the proposition, it is commonly held that in general adolescents are frequently non-compliant (Litt and Cuskey, 1980). It is clear, however, that adolescents challenge the ability of clinicians to engender good compliance and that the perjorative and judgemental labelling of young people as non-compliant is a completely unhelpful strategy for health care professionals.

Increasing the complexity of the asthma management plan is certain to decrease compliance. A balanced approach is required to ensure that the correct priorities are placed on the demands of the young person to avoid triggers, take medication, measure peak flow rates, keep diary cards and to take medication prior to exercise. Negotiating appropriate short-term goals with the young person about what is considered to be the current priority issue in their asthma management is an important strategy in avoiding the non-compliance associated with complex asthma management plans.

The problematic nature of compliance in young people is almost certainly related to a combination of cognitive and psychosocial developmental issues. The lack of a well developed sense of future time perspective limits the ability of a young person to modify their current behaviour in a way that they see is relevant to future health outcomes. Moreover, the emerging independence associated with adolescence quite understandably sees the young person experimenting with and making their own decisions about treatment plans. Understanding this perspective, enables physicians to adopt a risk minimization approach and avoid the adoption of threatening and critical attitudes.

A range of strategies needs to be drawn upon by the clinician to assist the young person in becoming compliant with treatment regimens. Such compliance promoting strategies include:

ensuring the treatment regimen is feasible and practical for the young person;

considering the acceptability of the treatment regimen to the young person's peers and friends;

consistently rewarding positive achievements even when deficits persist;

using a range of communication strategies including reminder telephone calls, cards, pamphlets and videos;

reference to the life experience of well known identities in the community with asthma who can act as role models;

developing simple reminder strategies, e.g. taping inhaler to toothbrush.

SPECIAL ISSUES FOR THE ADOLESCENT WITH ASTHMA

The body

Young people pay great attention to the growth and development of their bodies during adolescence. Concerns about bodily shape and appearance are common, particularly in young women. Adolescents are keen to know what side effects asthma medication will have, in particular how these side effects may affect their body image.

The impact of oral and inhaled corticosteroids on linear growth, adrenal function and bone metabolism are discussed elsewhere in this book. Notwithstanding the interest of adolescents in the general side effects of medication, it is likely that their immediate concern about steroid medication will be issues relating to body weight, facial appearance, hirsutism and acne. What may appear to be trivial and minor side effects in the eyes of clinicians can be devastating for the young person and account needs to be taken of this divergence of view when side effects are being considered.

Young women who have commenced menstruating may associate variations in asthma symptoms with their menstrual cycle. Although the impact of female sex hormones on respiratory physiology has been well studied (Dempsey et al, 1986), their impact on asthma control is less clear. It is appropriate to inquire about associations between variations in asthma symptoms and differing stages of the menstrual cycle. There is little data to inform a systematic therapeutic approach to such associations; however, it seems reasonable to explore individualized, preplanned variations in asthma medications during the menstrual cycle.

Educational settings and the impact of nocturnal asthma

Educational goals dominate the life of the late teenager. Academic performance is a major issue and the impact of asthma on school performance needs to be carefully explored by the clinician. Good communication with school professionals can greatly assist young people to manage their asthma better at school and to minimize the impact of asthma on academic achievement.

Nocturnal asthma disrupts sleep and contributes towards sleep fragmentation (Phillipson and Bowes, 1982). Fragmentation of sleep is closely associated with daytime sleepiness and decreased levels of alertness. The potential for unrecognized, and therefore poorly managed, nocturnal asthma to have an impact on academic achievement is considerable. The prudent use of long acting bronchodilators may be needed.

Occupational-related asthma is a significant issue in adults with asthma (Abramson et al, 1995). Young people making vocational choices may need to be advised about the potential impact of their chosen occupation on asthma symptoms and control.

Recreational settings and the impact of exercise-induced asthma

Exercise-induced asthma is commonly present in teenagers with asthma (Robertson et al, 1992). During adolescence young people develop their individual patterns of behaviour related to exercise. Some young people choose to be more competitive and intense about exercise and sport and the management of their exercise-induced asthma becomes a greater priority. Such young people need to be given adequate time and information to enable the development of effective preventive strategies for their exercise-induced symptoms. Clinicians need to be flexible and encourage experimentation with a variety of strategies including β_2-agonists, sodium chromoglycate or combinations of both. Frequently, young people forget to carry out an appropriate warm-up set of exercises prior to their competitive pursuits.

Other young people, released from the shackles of regular school physical education classes, adopt a more sedentary nonparticipatory approach to exercise. Indeed, the presence of asthma symptoms when exercise is undertaken may be used by the young person as an excuse for justifying their sedentary approach to life. Such young people need to be counselled about the positive health benefits that accrue from undertaking regular, aerobic exercise and encouraged to find ways to achieve this goal.

Scuba diving is a rapidly growing recreational pursuit that frequently attracts the interest of young people. Young people with asthma should not scuba dive and it is appropriate for clinicians to give early advice to adventure-seeking young people that encourages them to look at options other than scuba diving.

Recreational drug use

Young people commonly experiment with drugs during the teenage years, most commonly alcohol and tobacco. The prevalence of tobacco smoking in adults with asthma is the same as in adults without asthma (Abramson et al, 1992) and the same appears to be the case in adolescents (Robertson CF, personal communication). Preventing young people with asthma taking up smoking is of immense importance and a planned approach to this needs to be developed by clinicians caring for teenagers with asthma.

Tobacco is the most commonly smoked drug by teenagers and most young people are aware of the negative health impact of tobacco smoking on lung health. However, the negative health impact of marijuana smoking on lung health is less well understood by young people and needs to be reinforced. The use of volatile inhalants, e.g. 'glue sniffing' presents additional health risk to young people with asthma.

Transition to adult care

Paediatricians caring for young people with asthma need to plan for the transfer of clinical care to an adult physician. There is considerable potential for young people with asthma to simply fall down the gap that exists between paediatric and adult health care (Blum et al, 1993). Careful planning, including transition clinics, needs to occur to ensure continuity of quality care.

CONCLUSION

Adolescence is a time that presents a unique opportunity for the implementation of strategies that minimize the disease complications of asthma and promote good health. A programmed and systematic approach to the care of the young person with asthma during the teenage years enables the development of a sound foundation for the future good management of asthma throughout the adult years of life. To enable this to occur the clinician requires good communication skills and a clear understanding of the developmental and social issues impacting upon the life of young people with asthma.

SUMMARY

In addition to a good understanding of asthma management, the clinical care of the adolescent with asthma requires a good understanding of the processes of adolescence and how they interact with asthma and its treatment. Establishing good communication enables the development of mutually agreed upon goals of therapy. Specific compliance strategies informed by a knowledge of adolescent cognitive and psychosocial maturation need to be employed. Consideration needs to be given to how asthma impacts upon a young person in educational, recreational and vocational settings. Active interventions to prevent the uptake of tobacco smoking are important in promoting lung health. A dynamically changing approach to the care of the young person with asthma is required as they pass from the relatively dependent stages of childhood through to the relatively independent stage of adult life.

REFERENCES

Abramson M, Kutin J & Bowes G (1992) The prevalence of asthma in Victorian adults. *Australian and New Zealand Journal of Medicine* **22**: 358–365.

Abramson MJ, Kutin JJ, Rosier MJ & Bowes G (1995) Morbidity, medication and trigger factors in a community sample of adults with asthma. *The Medical Journal of Australia* **14**: 570–576.

Blum RW, Garell D, Hodgman CH et al (1993) Transition from child-centred to adult health care systems for adolescents with chronic conditions. *Journal of Adolescent Health* **14**: 570–576.

Dempsey JA, Olson EB & Skatrud JB (1986) Hormones and neurochemicals in the regulation of breathing. In Cherniack NS & Widdicombe JB (eds) *Handbook of Physiology, Section 3 Vol. 2 Control of Breathing*, pp 181–221.

Litt IF & Cuskey WR (1980) Compliance with medical regimens during adolescence. *Pediatric Clinics of North America* **27**: 3.

Phillipson EA & Bowes G (1982) Sleep disorders. In Fishman SP (ed.) *Update: Pulmonary Diseases and Disorders*, pp 256–273. New York: McGraw-Hill.

Robertson CF, Bishop J, Dalton M et al (1992) Prevalence of asthma in regional Victorian school children. *The Medical Journal of Australia* **156**: 831–833.

11

Psychological aspects of the management of asthma in children

SHEILA J. PARK

Since much of the lay public is said to view asthma as a primarily 'emotional' disease, clarity is required about when and how a mental health perspective can contribute to the well-being of children with asthma. A somatic predisposition is generally accepted, with bronchial hyper-irritability, an allergic propensity and autonomic reactivity as the basis. How these factors interact with emotional, environmental, familial and medical influences to determine the severity of the airway disease and the disability secondary to the asthma remains to be fully elucidated.

A review of studies (Isenberg et al, 1992) concluded that the empirical literature indicates that in about a third of asthmatics, psychological factors (including suggestion and emotional arousal) have an effect on airway tone, leading to increased airway obstruction. Expectations and emotions induced by factors known to the subject as likely to trigger asthma may potentiate the effect. Possible mechanisms include mediation via the vagus, and hyperventilation in response to stress causing bronchoconstriction by delivering cooler, drier air.

An immunological risk factor and a psychological risk factor, as measured by early parenting difficulties, are predictive of the onset of asthma in children with a genetically increased risk of developing the disease. The onset of asthma in a genetically vulnerable population can be delayed for at least a few years by careful attention to maternal stress levels in the years following the birth of the child (Mrazek et al, 1991).

Children with chronic illness, including asthma, have twice the rate of significant psychological adjustment problems (Cadman et al, 1987). Persistent functional disability and multiple medications are associated with an increased risk of emotional disturbance. Poor management of the condition and poor judgement of severity will affect the presentation, as will the child's experiences while occupying the sick role. Early trauma due to asthma itself and the effects of this on the parent–child interaction, parental childhood experiences including asthma, and the threat of loss of this or another child will predispose to anxiety in the family group during later occurring asthma episodes.

The complex interaction of these multidirectional elements, influencing the severity of the asthma itself and the associated behavioural and emotional disability, requires examination to assist the individual child and family and to extend our understanding of the illness.

Effects of the illness

The aim of treatment should be to limit disability and dysfunction directly attributable to the illness and to minimize secondary psychological and social handicaps. Sickness is a disruption which may lead to demoralization, fatigue, fear and alterations in self concept. Restriction of activities should be minimized in the intervals between attacks. Chronic illness may accelerate, delay or affect the adequacy of accomplishing normal developmental tasks and reduce resilience in the face of stressful life events.

Effects of treatment and hospital attendance

Systemic steroids may cause alterations in the body resulting in limitations of function. The secondary effects of reduced exercise tolerance may undermine the child's self esteem and possibly result in much poorer stress resistance, exercise being an important stress management activity. Retarded growth, altered body contour, acne and weight gain predispose to an altered body image and difficulties with the developmental challenges of adolescence. The prescription of steroids seems to have a powerful meaning for some children. In some it is anxiety relieving and hard to discontinue; in others it is associated with fear that the asthma is worse.

Regular emergency presentation may be a signal for a careful assessment to establish a more regular treatment regime, with optimal communication between general practitioners, specialists and the family. Where this is difficult to achieve it may be that mental health issues could usefully be investigated. If the child appears to be finding the sick role helpful in solving other difficulties, it is useful to help the child and family articulate the difficulties and generate solutions that address the underlying problem while allowing the child to function as normally as possible. Consultation with a mental health team may be considered.

Some writers refer to the advantages of a partnership between the child and the physician. While this may appear a useful approach, particularly if the parent is perceived as being a poor reader of the child's asthma, there exists a danger that the child is thereby encouraged to take premature responsibility. The child may become reliant for their sense of integrity on a belief that they can read their symptoms. Such a belief system about the severity of their asthma may be hard to alter. The parent and all other adults should be in partnership to assist the child.

Physician anxiety is inevitable, at times, when dealing with such a complex illness. Self awareness can be helpful in leading to consultation with a colleague.

The family

Interplaying with the asthma may be dysfunctions, including divorce, parental physical or psychiatric ill health, traumatic stresses affecting any or all family members, and financial worries. Most studies look predominantly at mothers but it is likely the variables involving fathers are equally interesting. In our unit fathers have, at times, had a major impact as a source of anxiety but also as a moderating force. Where the management of the child's condition is problematic, the family system as a whole requires careful consideration.

The school

The interaction between the school, the child and the family has potential for both positive and negative effects. Good basic information to schools should be automatic and in situations where potentially traumatic events are known to have occurred, the extreme example being where a child known to the school population has died of asthma, it may well be very constructive to offer more detailed support. Schools may be poorly equipped to cope with other than very straightforward asthma and an unhelpfully high anxiety may arise. An opportunity to improve knowledge accompanied by some discussion of fears and how to combat them may be offered.

The children themselves

Children at all levels of severity have been found to demonstrate problems of adjustment, suggesting that attention to psychological risk should not be limited to children with severe asthma (Perrin et al, 1989). The developmental stage of the child is always relevant. Pre-adolescents can be deceptively articulate; adolescents may have enormous difficulties taking advice. Difficulties with learning, or attention, may render school attendance less attractive than the sick role or may potentiate the level of stress caused by fear of the asthma.

In a study of 102 serial attenders at an asthma clinic (Weder et al, 1993), the lowest incidence of psychological risk factors was in those with only seasonal asthma. They found an increased rate in those with perennial and atypical asthma, Infection-induced asthma was associated with high levels of anxiety.

A review of the circumstances of children who had died during an asthma attack found that the risk was increased if the child had an emotional disturbance or if there was family dysfunction (Struck et al, 1985). While the risk was most acute for severe asthmatics there were rare cases where milder asthma had led to death. The child will be most in jeopardy when there is severe asthma, in an environment which has difficulties adapting to the illness and providing the child with appropriate support and structure.

ASTHMA, HYPERVENTILATION AND ANXIETY

Working in a hospital with primary, secondary and tertiary services available for children with asthma, we have identified a group which has caused much puzzlement and frustration. These patients are responding to a particular treatment approach, based on the formulation that panic anxiety is compounding the asthma presentation. They have in common a lack of correlation between objective lung function tests and their subjective experience of severity. It should be noted that the widely used Peak Flow Meter gives an effort-dependent result, so that these patients may not be recognized automatically by this method. A falsely low result may lead the child, family and physician, to whom the result has been reported, to conclude that the bronchospasm is worse than it is. Apparent better functioning when their attention is absorbed may contrast with increasingly frequent presentations despite the best endeavours of the physician. Some may be suffering side-effects of steroid medication to the concern of the physician who senses that this is out of step with the severity of the asthma. The impression is of a high level of anxiety in the family, although this is sometimes denied. The families are in a very worrying situation with the child never free from asthma and a belief that the asthma has entered a more serious phase.

All but one of 23 children, whose case histories we have reviewed, gave a history of a primary precipitating event which coincided with a perception that the asthma had worsened. The commonest was a traumatic, health-related experience, for example the child's awareness of the death of another child or witnessing of medical emergencies. Others were a major life event, such as the death of someone close, divorce, a house move, or major illness or accident in the family. In the case of four children, comments by adult authority figures such as doctors, nurses and teachers (often in the absence of a parent), were interpreted by the child as meaning their life was at risk. One 12-year-old girl was asked by a teacher if she was trying to kill herself by eating Burger Rings, which contain a synthetic colouring, and advised to talk to another girl whose cousin had died of asthma.

Deaths from asthma in the family or in people known to the children or parents were common, affecting more than a quarter, while a significant death among family and friends was recalled by three-quarters; the family of a 7-year-old girl had lost a baby to cot death 4 years earlier.

The histories were also characterized by multiple presentations and admissions, high medication use including steroids, loss of schooling and social contacts. Hyperventilation had been noted in about half. The peak age of presentation was 10–12 years with a range of 7–15 years. The histories revealed previous separation anxiety in a majority, and illness affecting family or friends, particularly parental mental illness, was prominent.

Apart from the frequency of the presentations, the physicians did not usually share the belief in a more sinister illness but were often becoming concerned at the high levels of medication which had been reached. At this stage a degree of panic had sometimes arisen in the child and family that the people on whom they depended for care did not understand the seriousness of the child's condition.

Theoretical basis for the treatment

The frequent presentations show a pattern which resembles that of panic disorder, with a traumatic experience from which there is apparent recovery. But when next there is an episode which suggests that asthma may be developing, there is a rapid deterioration of function. The next episode occurs quite soon thereafter and the intervals shorten rapidly to a point where the child and family have difficulty identifying periods when they believe the child to be well. A pattern may develop with rapid re-presentations very shortly after discharge. During this phase many different doctors may see the family, and medication levels may increase steeply.

Hyperventilation has been recognized as playing a part in the acute presentations of some asthmatics, including children. The dangers associated with undertreated asthma make it important to understand the way in which hyperventilation may complicate the picture as a preliminary to effective and safe treatment.

Hyperventilation, particularly the commoner but lesser known chronic variety, has been well described (Magarian, 1982; Brashear, 1983) as producing bodily symptoms which may be misconstrued by the patient and the physician as signifying physical illness, including asthma. In chronic hyperventilation, once hypocapnia has developed, the markedly reduced arterial blood carbon dioxide tension can be maintained with very little effort and only occasional deep breaths or sighs. This is important as clinical detection of hyperventilation cannot be relied on.

Hyperventilation has many causes including the physiological. Its role in the mediation of panic-anxiety disorder has been reviewed (Gelder, 1986). A cognitive component is a central part of panic, with the cognition or thought that the bodily sensations, which are the result of the hyperventilation, indicate serious physical illness.

The cognitive model of panic disorder (Clark, 1988) offers a way of understanding the interconnections between anxiety and asthma in children. Misinterpretation of the physiological, bodily effects of hyperventilation as evidence of physical illness (usually more severe asthma) may lead to fear of dying leading to a panic attack and further hyperventilation. The misinterpreted symptoms may include bodily sensations due to any cause, in the case of asthma these are likely to be breathing difficulties, chest or throat discomfort. However, there is nothing which precludes an asthma patient becoming afraid that they have heart disease when they notice palpitations or fearing they have a brain tumour when they experience headache, dizziness and some blurring of vision. Other symptoms of hyperventilation which are less well recognized include depersonalization (a feeling of being detached) which may lead to the person fearing they are going mad, and joint pains. The likelihood of any particular symptom being noticed will be influenced by recent experience.

Developmental changes lead to a mature concept of death emerging around 10–12 years. This makes the child particularly vulnerable to the stresses of chronic illness; an event which draws the child's attention to the possibility of death may cause a panic about personal mortality. Exposure to such events has been shown to act as a catalyst in speeding up this area of cognitive development (Reilly et al, 1983). Separation anxiety and school phobia are thought to be childhood equivalents of panic anxiety.

Treatment technique

A history is elicited from child and family giving particular attention to the aspects described above. An explanation is then offered about the possibility of confusing the symptoms of hyperventilation with the breathlessness of asthma. The physiological nature of hyperventilation is emphasized, with a description of how it might arise in the course of strenuous exercise but also how it is part of the experience of stress. A simple explanation of the evolutionary usefulness of the flight, fight or fright mechanism of the sympathetic nervous system can be rendered entertainingly, thus increasing the chances of the ideas being retained. The vicious circle which arises when the symptoms of anxiety are misunderstood is better comprehended when there is a clear statement that these are real bodily experiences, not imaginary ones. The relief engendered by this affirmation can then be linked to the statement that, although experienced in the body, these symptoms are in no sense evidence of serious physical disease and will certainly not lead to death. This is linked with the earlier history taking which should involve explicit enquiry about the child (and family) fearing death during some experiences.

Methods for escaping the vicious circle are then described with encouragement of the child to recall examples of times when their attention was distracted which seemed to result in improvement of their symptoms. The

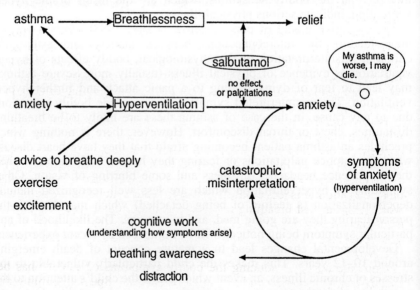

Figure 1.

suggestion is that a wide variety of distraction techniques may be helpful, including video games and watching television or self hypnosis, meditation and listening to music. If it works, use it! That the underlying aim is to slow the respiration rate to the automatic is clarified. It is comforting to some children and parents to realise that their bodies have an intrinsic respiration rate.

The suggestion is not to guess whether asthma or anxiety predominates, but to treat both. Figure 1 shows a diagram which may be offered to the child and family to take home and consider.

Some general principles

This pattern of hyperventilation occurs in children with mild, moderate and severe disease. Although consultation and referral will be necessary on occasion, the general principles of the intervention may be helpful when working with children with asthma as a whole. We have found it most effective, and we believe safest, to state clearly that the aim of treatment is to minimize secondary morbidity whether scholastic, social or pharmacological. Interestingly, we have seen considerable improvement in the degree of morbidity from the asthma. This may be related to the observation that, in some people, hyperventilation itself is a mechanism by which bronchospasm may be precipitated (Hibbert and Pilsbury, 1988).

Treating only the asthma may leave the child still hyperventilating which is then misconstrued as asthma which is unresponsive to treatment. Our aim is to teach asthmatics not to rely too heavily on their own judgement of severity but to simultaneously treat their bodily symptoms by attending to their asthma according to their physicians' instructions and to treat anxiety by non-noxious methods of cognitive work, breathing awareness and distraction techniques.

Children often already know how to distract their own attention by becoming absorbed in a game or a story. Some parents may also be able to move easily to this different way of responding once they realise that it is safe and indeed good treatment. To this point they may have become stuck in a watchful mode which has had the effect of maintaining anxiety in the family group.

Being clear that the mind and the body are part of an integrated organism will assist communication. Anyone with an asthma attack is bound to have concerns about their safety. 'It is not asthma' is likely to be construed by the patient as 'it is all in the mind'. The patient is experiencing bodily symptoms even though there may be no, or little bronchospasm detectable on auscultation. It is less confusing to say, 'Your symptoms are being made worse by your fast breathing rate. Lots of things can cause this, exercise, excitement or worries for example. The best way to treat it is to slow down your breathing. You cannot slow down your breathing too much; your body will see to that'.

Once the cycle of noticing the bodily symptoms of anxiety has been established, the source can be internal or external. Specific learning difficulties, particularly if not fully addressed may well make the prospect of a return to school stressful. Shyness and separation anxiety may be important. A conscientious or high achieving child may worry about how they will catch up after an absence. Where any of these problems are resistant to modification, consultation with a mental health professional at an early stage should be considered.

MUNCHAUSEN SYNDROME BY PROXY AND ASTHMA

A study of 1648 children presenting with asthma found management which constituted child abuse in 17 (1%). Ten were undertreated causing true asthma to become more serious, while in seven symptoms were fabricated, resulting in unnecessary investigations and procedures (Godding and Kruth, 1991).

Two cases in our practice illustrate the complexity and danger which may be present. A 12-year-old boy stopped having respiratory arrests only when his father finally dared to confide his wife's long history of physical investigations and operations, and her abuse of prescription drugs. The mechanism for the arrests seemed to be the induction of extremely high levels of anxiety in the boy, leading to hyperventilation and bronchospasm. It transpired that the mother had hyperventilated to the point of apnoea on many occasions. The father feared that if he acknowledged that his son's asthma was other than purely physical this would mean a future for his son like that of the mother.

In another case the pathological anxiety of the father, which led to him exaggerating the 8-year-old girl's symptoms, was made more problematic by the stepfather trying to negate the asthma completely. This left the child smothered in one setting and unprotected in the other. The respiratory arrests took place just after access to the smothering father, and in the ward following the departure of the parents who had been having a public row. The statutory welfare agency were informed so that the punitive stepfather could be assisted to understand the asthma better, allowing the mother to maintain more control over access to the father. There have been no further arrests and many fewer presentations to hospital with asthma.

Where such circumstances are suspected mental health consultation should be sought. Good communication between the primary physician and the specialist is crucial. Statutory intervention must be considered if there is not clear improvement and compliance with the regime instituted.

SUMMARY

A somatic predisposition interacts with psychological and social factors in a multidirectional manner to influence asthma itself and the associated behavioural and emotional disability. Mental health consultation should be an integral part of an asthma treatment service for children, and should be considered where there is:

  (i)   parental illness particularly asthma itself, psychosomatic difficulties, high anxiety or psychiatric difficulties;
 (ii)   frequent presentations to emergency;
(iii)   assumption of the sick role;
(iv)   loss of school and decreased social activity; and
 (v)   high usage of medication.

The interaction of panic anxiety with asthma should be suspected when the objective lung function tests are discrepant with the subjective complaints. A high index of suspicion is required if child abuse due to under- or overtreatment is to be detected and the child protected from a potentially fatal outcome.

Acknowledgements

The Thoracic Medicine Department of the Royal Children's Hospital and Dr. Daphne Glaun are acknowledged for their collaboration, support and encouragement.

REFERENCES

Brashear RE (1983) Hyperventilation syndrome. *Lung* **161:** 257–273.

Cadman D, Boyle M, Szatmari P & Offord DR (1987) Chronic illness disability and mental and social well-being. *Pediatrics* **79:** 805–813.

Clark DM (1988) A cognitive model of panic. In Rachman S & Maser JD (eds) *Panic: Psychological Perspectives*, p 31. Hillsdale NJ: Erlbaum.

Gelder MG (1986) Panic attacks: new approaches to an old problem. *British Journal of Psychiatry* **149:** 346–352.

Godding V & Kruth M (1991) Compliance with treatment in asthma and Munchausen by proxy. *Archives of Disease in Childhood* **66:** 956–960.

Hibbert G & Pilsbury D (1988) Demonstration and treatment of hyperventilation causing asthma. *British Journal of Psychiatry* **153:** 687–689.

Isenberg SA, Lehrer PM & Hochron S (1992) The effects of suggestion and emotional arousal on pulmonary function in asthma: a review and a hypothesis regarding vagal mediation. *Psychosomatic Medicine* **54:** 192–216.

Magarian GJ (1982) Hyperventilation syndromes: infrequently recognised common expressions of anxiety and stress. *Medicine* **61:** 219–236.

Mrazek DA, Klinnert M, Mrazek P & Macey T (1991) Early asthma onset: consideration of parenting issues. *Journal of the American Academy of Child and Adolescent Psychiatry* **30:** 277–282.

Perrin JM, MacLean WE & Perrin EC (1989) Parental perceptions of health status and psychologic adjustment of children with asthma. *Pediatrics* **83:** 26–30.

Reilly TP, Hasazi JE & Bond LA (1983) Children's conceptions of death and personal mortality. *Journal of Pediatric Psychology* **8:** 21–31.

Strunk RC, Mrazek DA, Wolfson GS & LaBrecque JF (1985) Physiological and Psychological characteristics associated with deaths from asthma in childhood: a case controlled study. *Journal of the American Medical Association* **254:** 1193–1198.

Weder M, Speck S, Spalinger J et al (1993) Psychosomatic symptoms in asthmatic children and adolescents. *Agents Actions Supplement* **40:** 27–37.

12

Patient, family and community education programmes for asthma

DANIEL M. HUGHES

As the prevalence of asthma has increased, so has public awareness with an increasing demand for information about the diagnosis, causes and treatment of this common condition.

Families of asthmatic children frequently seek information to help them understand their child's illness and how it might be treated successfully, and it is generally accepted that these families benefit from knowing more about asthma. Asthma education programmes that have measured asthma knowledge have shown that families not only learn more about the condition and its management but develop more confidence in their ability to manage asthma at home. What is far from clear is how much education of the child and family improves measurable asthma outcomes. Many asthma education programmes developed over the past 15 years have not been rigorously evaluated and have not been shown to be cost effective. Tacit acceptance of education interventions is no longer acceptable in the current economic climate and more rigour needs to be applied if we are to convince the 'payor' about the necessity and benefits of such programmes. It seems timely to address some of the issues surrounding patient, family and community education programmes for asthma.

Patient education is an essential part of routine health care and in the paediatric setting has been defined as any combination of planned learning experiences designed to facilitate adaptations of behaviour conducive to health (Nader, 1985). These behavioural changes may be carried out by the child, parent or other caregiver. By defining patient education in this way, it is clear that the desired outcome is behavioural change rather than the mere acquisition of knowledge.

Research in health education and compliance behaviour has led to the development of theories and models that may help us to understand behaviours observed in asthmatic children and their families (Bruhn, 1983). The social learning theory seems particularly attractive to health educators because it focuses on the interactions between the cognitive structures (what the patient thinks), the behaviour to be learned, and the physical and social environments (Nader, 1985). An asthma education programme which utilizes this theory would teach a child and family how to manage asthma by emphasizing self-efficacy or confidence in one's ability to

Baillière's Clinical Paediatrics—
Vol. 3, No. 2, May 1995
ISBN 0–7020–1986–0

perform behaviours designed to improve asthma control. This confidence would be gained by:

(a) mastering a difficult task such as recognizing asthma symptoms and taking appropriate medication;
(b) responding to verbal persuasion designed to encourage the desired behaviours;
(c) controlling physiological reactions particularly those that are stress-related; and
(d) appropriate modelling of behaviour such as the proper technique in using a metered dose inhaler (Nader, 1985).

If it is accepted that patient education is not only essential but should be defined in terms of behavioural changes that occur, it would be obvious that successful asthma management is more likely to occur if the child, or more often the child and family, initiate a series of actions designed to keep the symptoms of asthma under control. These actions may be short-term ones in the case of an acute asthma flareup, or long-term when there is a need for regular preventive therapy. The appropriate actions or behaviours necessary are most often, though not exclusively, learned during the family's encounter with some aspect of the health care system. It is here that behavioural science and patient education must come together to help families learn the skills and behaviours needed to manage asthma successfully. The term 'asthma self-management' has been used for this association between behaviour and education but it may not be the ideal one. It has been suggested that some physicians may feel excluded if they think the family is being taught to manage the child's asthma without their involvement, while parents may feel that they are being given sole responsibility for their child's asthma management and are ill-equipped to cope. Whether these concerns are valid or not, the focus should be shifted from the concept of 'self-management' to one of developing a 'partnership' between the family and the health professional. This may have the additional benefit of linking patient education with the child's medical care.

Asthma education programmes have flourished over the past 15 years and have been the subject of several conferences and entire journals (Fahey, 1981; Green et al, 1983; Sheffer and Buist, 1987; Sheffer, 1991, 1992). The best known programmes will be reviewed here.

The Open Airways Program (Clark et al, 1980; National Heart, Lung, and Blood Institute, 1984c; Clark et al, 1986) originated at Columbia University, New York and was developed with the needs of inner city, low income and low education families in mind. It is written in simple language and is available in Spanish. The program emphasizes communication with physicians and the interaction with the health care system as well as teaching decision-making and social skills. The programme uses a group dynamic process comprising 10–15 families where the topics of education sessions are based on actual experiences of the families. The programme can be offered to children aged 4–7 years and 8–14 years and consists of seven sessions of 60 minutes each. The curriculum was developed based on interviews with families designed to identify asthma-related management behaviours of parents. This programme was initially evaluted using 310 children (mean age 9 years) recruited from Allergy Clinics in four hospitals, and 85% were Black or Hispanic. The randomized controlled trial demonstrated improvements in both parental management and children's self-management behaviour. School performance declined in the control group, but both subjects and controls showed significant decrease in school absenteeism, and the difference between the decrease for subjects and controls was not significant. Decreases in health care use were observed only among children who had made use of health care facilities before the programme. This was probably due to the fact that many patients had mild asthma (86% of the patients had no baseline year hospitalizations and 38% made no baseline year emergency department visits). The study was completed with 175 subjects and 81 controls compared with 207 subjects and 103 controls at the outset, a significant drop-out rate. A cost analysis of the programme indicated that there were savings of $11.22 for emergency medical services for each $1 invested in programme costs.

Asthma Care Training (ACT) for kids (Lewis et al, 1984) was developed at the University of California in Los Angeles. This programme uses the car driving safety model with the traffic light analogy and is taught by nurses, teachers, or other health educators. The programme focuses on developing asthma management skills, improving general asthma knowledge and family dynamics, and consists of five sessions of 1 hour each. It is directed at children 8–12 years of age and has been evaluated in a randomized, controlled trial using 48 subjects and 28 controls followed for 12 months. The control group in this study received 4.5 hours of lecture presentations on asthma management. Both groups had equivalent increases in knowledge and beliefs about asthma, but the intervention group had increased self-reported compliance behaviour, fewer Emergency Department visits, and decreased hospitalization days with savings of $180 per year. This study also suffered from a significant drop-out rate with 31% of the controls and 23% of the intervention group dropping-out before the programme was completed.

The American Lung Association in Buffalo sponsored the Family Asthma Program (Hindi-Alexander and Cropp, 1981, 1984), a programme of six weekly sessions of 2 hours each directed at the 6–14 year age group. This programme consisted of a series of lectures, group discussion, physical exercises and was evaluated with a 1 year follow-up using 92 subjects but no controls. Pre- and post-test assessments showed a significant improvement in knowledge, health locus of control, and increased physical activities while school absenteeism decreased by 48%. There was no significant improvement in number of hospitalizations nor a statistically significant improvement in emergency visits.

Air Power (National Heart, Lung, and Blood Institute, 1984b; Wilson-Pessano and McNabb, 1985) was developed by from the American Institute of Research in Palo Alto, California. This programme consisted of four 1 hour sessions directed at the 9–13 age group. It teaches asthma self-management skills, provides asthma information, and instructions for relaxation exercises. Evaluation in 52 subjects showed an increase in the frequency of children's independent self-management behaviour as reported by parents but no change in any health outcome variables.

The Air Wise Program (National Heart, Lung, and Blood Institute, 1984a; McNabb et al, 1985) is similar to the Air Power Program but consists of four to six hourly sessions with one-on-one teaching designed to target the child with difficult to manage asthma. The programme is tailored to meet the needs of severe cases and individual discussions and explanations are given to each child based on the child's particular needs. This programme was evaluated in a randomized controlled trial in two small studies, and demonstrated a decrease in the number of emergency visits, but no statistical tests of significance were provided. Estimated cost savings of about $507 per year per child were gained after subtracting programme costs. Non-emergency visits and medical requirements did not differ between groups before and after the intervention (McNabb et al, 1985).

The Children's Asthma Research Institute and Hospital in Denver developed the Living with Asthma Program (Creer and Leung, 1981; National Heart, Lung, and Blood Institute, 1985) consisting of eight weekly sessions of 1 hour each, targetting the 8–13 years group. It emphasized the need to promote developmentally appropriate self-management skills. The focus of the programme is on family dynamics and the application of social learning techniques for developing asthma management skills. Short-term evaluation of this programme showed improvement in asthma management knowledge and attitudes, while long-term follow-up, carried out after the original control group had received the programme, showed better peak expiratory flow rates and lower school absenteeism rates. No data on hospitalizations or emergency department use were provided.

The Pittsburgh Program (Fireman et al, 1981) consists of six sessions, 1–2 hours each, in both a group and individual format. The programme is directed to a younger age group, ages 2–14 years, in an office setting. Four sessions consist of individual instruction and two are group sessions. Using a nurse educator with phone follow-up, the programme was evaluated in a randomized controlled trial using 13 subjects and 13 controls. There were fewer hospitalizations and emergency department visits in the intervention group along with a decrease in school absenteeism and in frequency of asthma attacks. No baseline pretreatment data were collected and knowledge of asthma was not studied. No information was available on the individual programme provided by the nurse.

Superstuff (Weiss, 1981; Rakos et al, 1985) is a self-administered programme developed for the American Lung Association. It consists of a self-contained teaching kit with separate components for parents and children and is regarded as a true self-sufficient instructional unit with no direct teacher involvement. The programme has an unlimited number of sessions given at any time on an individualized format designed for children of ages 6–12 years. This programme has been evaluated in a randomized controlled trial using 20 subjects and 23 controls and demonstrated increased children self-reports of asthma self-control skills but no decrease in emergency visits or school absenteeism.

An interactive computer game entitled 'Asthma Command' (Rubin et al, 1986) has been developed to teach strategies for coping with asthma symptoms. This program consists of six sessions of approximately 45 minutes each, directed at the 7–12 year olds. The programme was evaluated using 25 subjects and 29 controls, demonstrating an increase in knowledge about asthma, with subjects reporting more appropriate behaviour regarding asthma management. No significant differences were found in visits to physicians, emergency department visits, or number of hospitalizations.

A preschool programme for the 2–5 year age group has been developed by the American Lung Association of Utah and the University of Utah. The Self Care Rehabilitation Program in Pediatric Asthma (Whitman et al, 1985) consists of six 1 hour classes for parents and children with the parents present only in the first and last session. In addition, another programme is available for children age 6–14 years involving eight 90 minute classes for parents and children. The programme provides information and teaches skills for managing asthma along with physical conditioning. The programme was evaluated in 38 school-age children for 3 months and showed improvement in knowledge and self-management skills. Twenty-one preschool children followed for 3 months showed a decrease in the number of episodes of asthma.

Two programmes have been designed for the school setting. Open Airways for the School (Kaplan et al, 1986; Evans et al, 1987a) focuses on children 8–11 years of age and consists of six 1 hour educational sessions. The parents do not take part initially but are involved in the children's homework assignments. In a 1 year follow-up the active group improved compared to the control group in academic performance and asthma self-management behaviours. Teaching Myself About Asthma (Parcel et al, 1979, 1980) is a second programme offered for schools targeting the 6–12 year age group as well as encouraging home participation by parents. This is a lengthy course consisting of 24 weekly sessions of 40 minutes each given by teachers, school psychologists and nurses. Evaluation of this programme showed that children developed greater feelings of control over their asthma as well as having less anxiety. Medical outcomes were not significantly changed, and the authors attributed this to the fact that the individual medical needs of the children could not be addressed and recommended that medical care and education must be linked (Parcel et al, 1980).

STRENGTHS OF THE PROGRAMMES

The asthma education programmes reviewed have a number of features in common. Most target the 6–14 year age group and their parents, delivering general asthma knowledge to a literate audience. Exceptions are the Air Wise Program (National Heart, Lung, and Blood Institute, 1984a) designed for individualized instruction, Open Airways (National Heart, Lung, and Blood Institute, 1984c) directed to a low income, inner city population, and the Self Care Rehabilitation Program in paediatric asthma (Whitman et al, 1985) for the preschool group. Usually eight to 12 families meet for 1–2 months with parents and children generally meeting both separately and together in a group format, instructed by a variety of asthma educators trained for the purpose. Superstuff (Weiss, 1981) is the exception, being a self-administered take home programme. Programmes tend to be clinic-based and two have been adapted to the school setting: Teaching Myself About Asthma (Parcel et al, 1979, 1980) and Open Airways (Kaplan et al, 1986; Evans et al, 1987a). Where details of the programmes are available, the curricula tend to be fairly uniform and programmes encourage a partnership approach with the child's physician. On the whole, asthma self-management programmes have been shown to increase the participants' knowledge of asthma along with increasing the reported use of self-management behaviours. Recipients express increased confidence and improved self-esteem as well as gaining new coping strategies. The group format has the added advantage of allowing families to share experiences and learn from one another.

WEAKNESSES OF THE PROGRAMMES

The asthma education programmes described here as well as other pro-grammes have been extensively reviewed and the deficiencies are gener-ally known (Popham and Yalow, 1983; Thoresen and Kirmil-Gray, 1983; Wilson, 1983; Evans et al, 1987b; Klingelhofer, 1987; Howland et al, 1988; Klingelhofer and Gershwin, 1988). The development of future asthma education programmes should not proceed without an awareness of existing programme deficiencies and the design of strategies to over-come them.

Rarely do evaluations of education programmes provide any information about the functional severity of asthma and the subjects mostly reflect the severity of asthma in the childhood population, the majority being mild (Rosier et al, 1994). Sample sizes have often been insufficient and studies have lacked the power to show significant differences in outcome measures. Likewise, the behavioural diversity of subjects has not been defined in the various programmes and this issue awaits further study. Education programmes have been based in clinics, offices, homes, schools, summer camps, and institutions, and there is little information available to indicate that they can be transferred successfully beyond the setting in which they were studied. A programme developed for a hospital-based tertiary care respiratory clinic is unlikely to be suitable for a primary care practice in a rural community. Health care institution programmes tend to be physician-focused and may be more costly to run while those based in the community are more consumer-oriented and less costly. It has also been suggested that community-based programmes are less likely to encourage dependency on the medical care system (Mullen and Mullen, 1983). Sufficient information on the structure and content of programmes must be provided to allow for replication by others particularly in different settings. Duration of the instruction has varied from 3 to 24 hours with target populations varying in age from 2 to 19 years, making inter-group and inter-programme comparisons difficult. The majority of the programmes have been developed for the school-aged child with few programmes designed for preschoolers, although a programme is currently being developed to address the specific problems of this population (Wilson et al, 1993). It is also rare that programmes have recognized the different developmental levels of children and incorporate the necessary content and strategies (Howell et al, 1992).

Rarely is information provided on the asthma educators themselves. This information is essential particularly in situations where it seems that the enthusiasm and commitment of the educators is the determining factor in a programme's success rather than the programme itself (Popham and Yalow, 1983). In some studies, control groups have not been used and where they do exist the comparability of control and intervention groups has not always been established. Besides an appropriate baseline analysis the outcomes resulting from the intervention must be clearly defined, especially for a condition such as asthma that can be so variable from one season to another and often improves with age. Baseline measures are not always reported and follow-up has rarely been for longer than 12 months making long-term benefits impossible to assess. In some cases outcome measures showed no improvement or the degree of improvement did not reach statistical significance, small sample size occasionally being the reason. Sources of data for outcome measures such as school absenteeism and days in hospital have sometimes relied on parental recall rather than school or hospital records. Reliable data on school absenteeism because of asthma, physician and emergency department acute care visits, hospitalizations, and number of days hospitalized must be provided.

Instruments for assessing asthma knowledge are rarely criterion-based, and there is no evidence to show that the increase in knowledge obtained following the intervention is educationally significant. Programmes that do not have a link with the child's medical management make it difficult to determine whether a positive outcome is due to the programme intervention or a change in the child's medical treatment programme. The child's medical treatments should be determined and recorded. The investigators should ensure that all children are receiving appropriate and sufficient therapies before embarking on the education programme. A potentially beneficial programme may be overshadowed by a child's poor medical management.

In spite of what is known about behavioural strategies for self-management programmes, rarely is the psychology of self-managed change applied to childhood asthma programmes (Thoresen and Kirmil-Gray, 1983). Programme developers must recognize that passive transfer of knowledge is not sufficient. The goal is to change behaviour with resulting improvement in the child's asthma control leading to defined, clinically significant outcomes. A programme that fails to change asthma management behaviours is unlikely to succeed. The evaluation, or more often the lack of evaluation, of asthma self-management programmes has been previously reviewed (Popham and Yalow, 1983; Wilson, 1983). Programme evaluations that have a research orientation tend to focus on proving or disproving a programme's worth and survival of the programme may

depend on the results. The majority of asthma self-management programmes have used this approach. A more appropriate evaluation instrument would be one designed to be used during a programme's execution to
produce information useful for quality improvement.

Attrition is a significant problem in some programmes and has not been
well studied to date. While it is important to know why some families drop
out, it may be equally important to know the characteristics of those
families that remain. There is the possibility that the benefits of the
programme have more to do with their own personal attributes than the
programme itself. It has been suggested that those who remain in the programmes are not typical of the normal population (Klingelhofer and
Gershwin, 1988). Shrinking health care budgets make it mandatory that all
programmes be cost-effective but with few exceptions most studies have
not provided this important information (Krahn, 1994).

BARRIERS TO PROGRAMME DEVELOPMENT

Many barriers impede the development and successful implementation of
asthma self-management programmes. These barriers can include health
care system factors, physical resource issues, patient/family issues, and
health care professional/educator factors (Mullen and Mullen, 1983;
Klingelhofer, 1987; Parker et al, 1989).

Health care system

A technology-oriented health care system is a major barrier to implementing education programmes. Many systems are focused on what needs to be
'done' to a patient rather than learned by the patient and family.
Reimbursement programmes, particularly for hospital-based care, reward
acute care encounters and procedural activities but are often not sympathetic to preventive or educational interventions. Funds to establish and
maintain a self-management programme may be difficult to obtain where
such attitudes exist. A significant number of patients receive their medical
care, usually at the time of crises, from emergency departments, out-patient
clinics, and walk-in clinics rather than from their primary physician.
Communication is often unsatisfactory and the continuity of care is poor.
Families frequently come away from such encounters confused by the
inconsistencies in asthma management. In addition, some aspects of the
health care system seem to be directed more to meeting the needs of those
working in the system rather than in meeting the needs of the patients.
Some education programmes are stand-alone programmes not always
linked to the medical management of the individual and concentrating
mainly on the passive transfer of information.

Physical resources

Most physicians' offices or hospital clinics do not have sufficient space

available for group educational sessions and most busy emergency departments have neither the time, staff, or inclination to get involved in asthma
education practices beyond the provision of written material that the family
can take to read at a more opportune time. A cursory review of some of the
abundant reading material available on asthma will reveal inconsistencies
that can be confusing to families. The readability level of some material
exceeds the level of the population to which it is directed and may not be
linguistically or culturally appropriate. Families may become confused
when the information in a pamphlet differs from what they have been told
by the physician or some other health educator.

Patient/family

Families that are not convinced about the need for education are unlikely to
persevere with a programme, particularly a lengthy one. This is more likely
when the child has trivial asthma or when the parents and/or child have
underestimated the severity of the child's asthma. Worry about medication
side effects should also not be underestimated, and this problem may
continue to grow with the increased use and occasional abuse of inhaled
steroids in children. Concerns need to be discussed fully with families to
ensure that any reluctance to use medication is addressed. Communication
problems between families and health care professionals can detract from
the benefits that might be gained from asthma education programmes. The
intimidation felt by some parents during even routine health care visits may
be just one factor. Conflicting schedules, making suitable travel or child
care arrangements, the trend for some parents to have more than one job,
single parent families, children living with separated parents in two different households are just a few of the problems that seem to be increasing and
can act as barriers. Some families may have problems in complying with
advice given in an educational programme because of their inability to pay
for asthma medications, particularly the more expensive anti-inflammatory
agents, the difficulty in avoiding some triggers especially perfumes and
cigarette smoke in public places, and the need to use daycare arrangements
involving large numbers of children and subsequent exposure to viral
infections.

Health care professionals/educators

Most physicians receive little training in behavioural strategies that are
useful for asthma management or skill development needed to be a good
teacher—both essentials for asthma self-management programmes.
Without an interested, motivated, and knowledgeable physician who is
prepared to spend more than the usual 10 minute office visit, a self-
management programme or any educational endeavour that depends on
direct physician involvement is unlikely to be successful. Even when the
physician is not directly involved in the programme, his or her commitment
and support is still required. A physician who feels threatened by the idea

of asthma self-management or of developing a partnership with a family to manage the child's asthma can quickly undermine what otherwise might be a successful programme (Parker et al, 1989). If there is no linkage between the education programme and the medical management, the programme is unlikely to meet its objectives. Likewise, the enthusiasm, knowledge, and commitment of other health professionals and educators in developing and sustaining a self-management programme are essential for programme success.

PROGRAMME DEVELOPMENT

Considering the existing barriers that must be overcome as well as the deficiencies of many of the current asthma self-management programmes, developing a successful, effective education programme is not a small task. The Air Power and Open Airways Programs were developed only after a detailed assessment of existing knowledge, attitudes, and behaviours as well as determining the information and skills children and the caretakers required, to ensure a successful outcome. Collaboration should include individuals knowledgeable in medicine, behavioural sciences, and education. Families come to such programmes with very different levels of knowledge, skills, fears, misconceptions, and experiences with asthma, both good and bad. The education programme, in addition to its general components, should offer individualized attention to deal with these differences.

Key to the successful implementation of an asthma education programme is the selection and training of appropriate individuals to conduct the programme (Clark et al, 1993). The average nurse, respiratory therapist, or community volunteer does not possess sufficient knowledge of asthma, behavioural management techniques, or of group dynamics, and formal training should be required of such individuals. Training programmes with appropriate certification are sparse and should be developed. Probably the best known is the Asthma Training Centre mainly for practice-nurses working in the National Health Service in the United Kingdom (Cote et al, 1994).

Programme curriculum

Table 1 provides a list of the major topics that should be covered in an education programme. Families benefit from understanding the basics of the pathophysiology of asthma, including the mechanisms of airways obstruction as well as the symptoms and common triggers. Knowledge of the individual child's triggers is essential if avoidance measures are to be undertaken. The most confusing aspect of asthma management for families (and some health professionals) is the distinction between medications designed to prevent asthma symptoms (anti-inflammatories or preventives) and those for symptom relief (bronchodilators or relievers). There is a need for clearly written instructions (literacy assumed) for managing an asthma

Table 1. Content for asthma education programme.

1.	Basic pathophysiology
2.	Symptoms
3.	Triggers
4.	Treatments
	non medical
	medical
5.	Asthma medications
	preventers/relievers
	side effects
6.	Action plan
7.	Monitoring
8.	Seeking medical attention
9.	Exercise induced asthma symptoms
10.	Asthma and school

flare-up. The Action Plan may include use of a peak flow meter for selected cases. Parents occasionally express concern about their inability to determine when they should bring their child to medical attention during an asthma exacerbation. This, together with the tendency for some teenagers with asthma to ignore worsening asthma symptoms, requires full discussion since under-recognition and under-appreciation of the severity of an asthma attack has been linked to asthma deaths (British Thoracic Association, 1982). Parents need guidance and support for dealing with school personnel concerning their asthmatic child, deficiencies having been well documented (Freudenberg et al, 1980). Satisfactory knowledge of such a curriculum is not sufficient and specific behavioural strategies need to be taught to allow families to use their knowledge to improve the child's asthma control.

Physicians' role

Considering that most patient education is carried out in the physician's office, what might the individual physician do to try to ensure successful asthma outcomes. The first priority is to get the child's current symptoms under control. This is best done during the first health care encounter and requires reviewing and where necessary altering the child's medical management. The successful reduction of the child's asthma symptoms sends two important messages to the family: (1) that asthma symptoms can be brought under control; and (2) that the physician needs to work with the family to accomplish this—the first step in the partnership process. Education about the diagnosis of asthma itself is critical. It has been clearly shown that the diagnostic label affects whether the wheezy child will be treated with antibiotics or bronchodilators and whether appropriate explanations are given (Anderson et al, 1981; Speight et al, 1983). From the outset the physician must appreciate that it is the child and the family that manage the child's asthma using the information and tools provided by the physician or other health professionals. Most decision making in asthma management occurs away from the physician's office and the hospital. Both family and physician need to understand that successful asthma management requires an effective working relationship. Asthma education is not simply a one way transfer of information, and families need time to ask questions and discuss their worries. The physician can send an important signal to a family that he is prepared for such discussion by asking open ended questions like, 'Some parents worry about side effects from medications or that their child might die from asthma, what do you worry about?' Translating knowledge of asthma into specific behaviours requires some familiarity with the subject of compliance (Sackett and Haynes, 1976). The physician should incorporate into the management programme specific strategies for improving compliance such as:

(a)   developing a satisfactory relationship and two way communication that will enable the family to develop confidence in the physician;
(b)   keeping the treatment regimens as simple as possible;
(c)   providing clearly written instructions including an action plan for managing acute exacerbations;
(d)   providing continuity of care; and
(e)   providing consistent accurate information (Klingelhofer, 1987).

The physician should set realistic goals for the child and be prepared to accept that the child's goals may differ from those of the physician. A teenager with asthma is more likely to comply with a particular therapeutic regimen if he can see some relevant benefits and his goals are being met. Like the child's medical regimen, the family's education needs to be individualized according to the particular needs. When required, the physician must be prepared to alter the direction of these efforts and appreciate that there will be occasions when additional help may be required, e.g. community health nurse home visit, phone call follow-up, or additional educational material. Families respond favourably to compliments about their management abilities, and opportunities for positive reinforcement should never be missed. If the physician is either unwilling or unable to spend the time necessary to educate the child and family about asthma management, this task should be delegated to another. This may require expanding the role of the office or clinic nurse, or referring the family to a community asthma programme. If the latter option is chosen, the physician should ensure that the programme content is consistent with the advice that he is giving the family. Parents are very quick to note inconsistencies in the messages given by different health professionals. From the perspective of the community itself, the physician, if not actually involved in a particular education programme, should at least be prepared to act as a resource person. Asthma education programmes working in isolation are unlikely to be successful and a close link with a medical practitioner is essential.

FUTURE RESEARCH

It should be apparent that asthma education programmes require more study (Mullen and Mullen, 1983; Parker, 1987; Clark et al, 1993). Some of the key areas are: benefits of individual versus group programmes, compliance with therapeutic regimens, attrition rates, tools, outcome measures, targetting specific groups, and cost effectiveness of programmes. Programmes for pre-schoolers need to be developed. Training requirements for asthma educators should be established and more information is needed on physician knowledge and practice.

In an attempt to reduce the morbidity associated with childhood asthma, self-management asthma programmes have been developed. Although these programmes can improve knowledge of asthma and increase asthma self-management behaviour, their impact on asthma morbidity has yet to be proven to the extent that any particular programme can be endorsed. The task of educating families of asthmatic children still rests largely with the individual physician, subject to the various inherent difficulties mentioned.

SUMMARY

Numerous asthma education programmes directed to children and their families have been developed over the past 15 years. The main objective of these programmes, either implicit or stated, is to improve knowledge of asthma and its management with a reduction in morbidity and mortality. Asthma self-management education programmes have attempted to meet these objectives by combining educational and behavioural strategies and encouraging a partnership approach between the health professional and family. That these programmes have not been widely accepted may be in part due to the failure to provide convincing evidence that the outcomes justify the expense and effort. The development of successful asthma education programmes is hindered by barriers such as a technology-oriented health care system, limited physical and human resources, limited access for some families, and the hesitation of some physicians. Well intentioned but inadequately trained health educators can also impede a programme's success. Most asthma education will continue to be delivered in physicians' offices although this is still not ideal. Those wishing to develop asthma education programmes should be aware of the deficiencies of existing programmes and the barriers that will be encountered. Much research remains to be done before achieving the ideal programme.

REFERENCES

Anderson HR, Bailey PA, Cooper JS & Palmer JC (1981) Influence of morbidity, illness label and social, family, and health service factors on drug treatment of childhood asthma. *Lancet* **ii:** 1030–1032.

British Thoracic Association (1982) Death from asthma in two regions of England. *British Medical Journal* **285:** 1251–1255.

Bruhn JG (1983) The application of theory in childhood asthma self-help programs. *Journal of Allergy and Clinical Immunology* **72:** 561–577.

Clark NM, Gotsch A & Rosenstock IR (1993) Patient, professional, and public education on behavioral aspects of asthma: A review of strategies for change and needed research. *Journal of Asthma* **30:** 241–255.

Clark NM, Feldman CH, Freudenberg N et al (1980) Developing education for children with asthma through study of self-management behavior. *Health Education Quarterly* **7:** 278–297.

Clark NM, Feldman CH, Evans D et al (1986) The impact of health education on frequency and cost of health care use by low income children with asthma. *Journal of Allergy and Clinical Immunology* **78:** 108–115.

Cote J, Golding J, Barnes G & Boulet L-P (1994) Educating the educators—how to improve teaching about asthma. *Chest* **106:** S242–247.

Creer T & Leung P (1981) The development and evaluation of a self-management program for children with asthma. In Fahey JL (ed.) *Self-management Educational Programs for Childhood Asthma*, Los Angeles: University of California.

Evans D, Clark NM, Feldman CH et al (1987a) A school health education program for children with asthma ages 8–11. *Health Education Quarterly* **14:** 267–279.

Evans D, Clark NM & Feldman CH (1987b) School health education programs for asthma. *Clinical Reviews in Allergy* **5:** 207–212.

Fahey JL (Conference Chairman) (1981) *Self-management education programs for childhood asthma*. University of California, Los Angeles.

Fireman P, Friday GA, Gira C et al (1981) Teaching self-management skills to asthmatic children and their parents in an ambulatory care setting. *Pediatrics* **68:** 341–348.

Freudenberg N, Feldman CH, Clark NM et al (1980) The impact of bronchial asthma on school attendance and performance. *Journal of School Health* **50:** 522–526.

Green LW, Goldstein RA, Parker SR (eds) (1983) Workshop Proceedings on self-management of childhood asthma. *Journal of Allergy and Clinical Immunology* **72(5) Part 2:** 519–626.

Hindi-Alexander M & Cropp GJA (1981) Community and family programs for children with asthma. *Annals of Allergy* **46:** 143–148.

Hindi-Alexander M & Cropp GJA (1984) Evaluation of a family asthma program. *Journal of Allergy and Clinical Immunology* **74:** 505–510.

Howell JH, Flaim T & Lung CL (1992) Patient education. *Pediatric Clinics of North America* **39:** 1343–1361.

Howland J, Bauchner H & Adair R (1988) The impact of pediatric asthma education on morbidity. *Chest* **94:** 964–969.

Kaplan DL, Rips JL, Clark NM et al (1986) Transferring a clinic based health education program for children with asthma to a school setting. *Journal of School Health* **56:** 267–271.

Klingelhofer EL (1987) Compliance with medical regimens, self-management programs, and self-care in childhood asthma. *Clinical Reviews in Allergy* **5:** 231–247.

Klingelhofer EL & Gershwin ME (1988) Asthma self-management programs: Premises, not promises. *Journal of Asthma* **25:** 89–101.

Krahn M (1994) Issues in the cost-effectiveness of asthma education. *Chest* **106:** S264–269.

Lewis CE, Rachelefsky G, Lewis MA et al (1984) A randomized trial of A.C.T (Asthma Care Training) for kids. *Pediatrics* **74:** 478–486.

McNabb WL, Wilson-Pessano SR, Hughes GW & Scamagas P (1985) Self-management education of children with asthma: Air Wise. *American Journal of Public Health* **75:** 1219–1220.

Mullen PD & Mullen LR (1983) Implementing asthma self-management education in medical care settings—issues and strategies. *Journal of Allergy and Clinical Immunology* **72:** 611–622.

Nader PR (1985) Improving the practice of pediatric patient education: A synthesis and selective review. *Preventive Medicine* **14:** 688–701.

National Heart, Lung, and Blood Institute (1984a) *Air Wise: Self-management of asthma through individual education*. Bethesda MD: NIH Publication no. 84-2363.

National Heart, Lung, and Blood Institute (1984b) *Air Power: Self-management of asthma through group education*. Bethesda MD: NIH Publication no. 85-2362.

National Heart, Lung, and Blood Institute (1984c) *Open Airways/Respiro Abierto: Asthma self-management program*. Bethesda MD: NIH Publication no. 84-2635.

National Heart, Lung, and Blood Institute (1985) *Living with asthma—Part I Manual for teaching parents the self-management of childhood asthma; Part II Manual for teaching children the self-management of asthma*. Bethesda MD: NIH Publication no. 85-2364.

Parcel GS, Nader PR & Tiernan K (1980) A health education program for children with asthma. *Journal of Developmental and Behavioral Pediatrics* **1:** 128–132.

Parcel GS, Tiernan K, Nader PR & Weiner L (1979) *Teaching Myself about Asthma*, St. Louis: CV Mosby.

Parker SR (1987) The future role of asthma self-management. *Journal of Allergy and Clinical Immunology* **80:** 511–514.

Parker SR, Mellins RB & Sogn S (1989) Asthma education: A national strategy. *American Review of Respiratory Disease* **140:** 848–853.

Popham WJ & Yalow ES (1983) Methodologic problems in the evaluation of self-management programs. *Journal of Allergy and Clinical Immunology* **72:** 581–590.

Rakos RF, Grodek MV & Mach KK (1985) The impact of a self-administered behavioral program on pediatric asthma. *Journal of Psychosomatic Research* **29:** 101–108.

Rosier MJ, Bishop J, Nolan T et al (1994) Measurement of functional severity of asthma in children. *American Journal of Respiratory and Critical Care Medicine* **149:** 1434–1441.

Rubin DH, Leventhal JM, Sadock RT et al (1986) Educational intervention by computer in childhood asthma: A randomized clinical trial testing the use of a new teaching intervention in childhood asthma. *Pediatrics* **77:** 1–10.

Sackett DL & Haynes RB (eds) (1976) *Compliance with Therapeutic Regimens* Baltimore: John Hopkins University Press.

Sheffer AL (1991) Guidelines for the diagnosis and management of asthma. *Journal of Allergy and Clinical Immunology* **88(3) Part 2:** 425–534.

Sheffer AL (1992) *International Consensus Report on Diagnosis and Treatment of Asthma.* National Heart, Lung, and Blood Institute. Bethesda MD: NIH Publication no. 92-3091.

Sheffer AL & Buist AS (eds) (1987) Proceedings of the asthma mortality task force. *Journal of Allergy and Clinical Immunology* **80(3) Part 2:** 361–514.

Speight ANP, Lee DA & Hey EN (1983) Underdiagnosis and undertreatment of asthma in childhood. *British Medical Journal* **286:** 1253–1256.

Thoresen CE & Kirmil-Gray K (1983) Self-management psychology and the treatment of childhood asthma. *Journal of Allergy and Clinical Immunology* **72:** 596–606.

Weiss J (1981) Superstuff: An asthma self-management training program developed for the American Lung Association. In Fahey JL (ed.) *Self-management Educational Programs for Childhood Asthma.* **2:** 273–294. Bethesda MD: National Institute of Allergy and Infectious Diseases.

Whitman N, West D, Brough F & Welch M (1985) A study of a self-care rehabilitation program in pediatric asthma. *Health Education Quarterly* **12:** 333–342.

Wilson S, Starr-Schneidkraut NJ, Austin DM et al (1993) Early intervention with parents of very young children with asthma reduces nocturnal symptoms and improves overall control. *American Review of Respiratory Diseases* **147 (supplement 4):** A774.

Wilson SR (1983) Response: Methodologic problems in the evaluation of self-management programs. *Journal of Allergy and Clinical Immunology* **72:** 590–595.

Wilson-Pessano SR & McNabb WL (1985) The role of patient education in the management of childhood asthma. *Preventive Medicine* **14:** 670–687.

Index

Note: Page numbers of article titles are in **bold** type.